SHAPEDOWN®

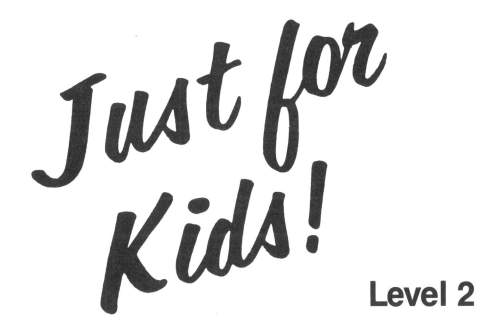

Level 2

Laurel M. Mellin, M.A., R.D.

University of California, San Francisco

Balboa Publishing · San Anselmo, CA

The development of this SHAPEDOWN Children's Workbook was supported in part by the Department of Family and Community Medicine and the John Tung/American Cancer Society Clinical Nutrition Education Center, School of Medicine, University of California, San Francisco. Developmental testing of this workbook was facilitated by the Department of Pediatrics of the University.

The development of this workbook was based on the experience and perspectives of many health professionals and parents. We are particularly grateful for the contributions of Marna Cohen, M.S.W., Lisa Frost, P.N.P., M.N.S., and Carl Greenberg, M.S., and the support of Donald L. Fink, M.D., Interim Chair, Department of Family and Community Medicine.

Use of this workbook is restricted to participants in licensed SHAPEDOWN Weight Management Programs conducted by health professionals who function in interdisciplinary teams, have completed required technical training and maintain membership in The Center For Adolescent Obesity.

Reviewers are requested to obtain complete program materials from Balboa Publishing at the address below.

Copyright 1988 by Laurel M. Mellin

Second revised edition

Printed in the United States of America

**Library of Congress
Cataloging in Publication Data**
Mellin, Laurel M.

SHAPEDOWN Just for Kids!
Level Two Workbook

Library of Congress Catalog
Card No.: 88-70316
ISBN 0-935902-16-3 Paperback

Illustrations: Martha Weston
Graphic design: Leadfeather Graphics
Typography: ProType Graphics, Inc.

Published by: **Balboa Publishing**
            11 Library Place
            San Anselmo, CA 94960
            (415) 453-8886

CONTENTS

1. CINDY AND THE CLOWN'S SURPRISE

In the back of Ms. Bacon's classroom was a cozy corner. Kids lucky enough to have their desks in that corner of room 6 were out of earshot of Ms. Bacon. These four kids could whisper, tell riddles and giggle without Ms. Bacon hearing a sound. It was the middle of the year now and they were quite experienced at carefully slipping a note—with a special secret scribble in code—from desk to desk until it reached the boy or girl whose name was carefully lettered on it.

This morning Ms. Bacon had a terrible headache that she got from worrying about her bird, Meredith, who was expecting baby birds any moment. You see, Meredith had been sitting on those eggs for so many days that Ms. Bacon was afraid that they were empty. Today she had to take the eggs to the vet to find out whether the five eggs were baby birds . . . or not.

Ms. Bacon wanted peace and quiet to nurse her headache and think about her bird. With her eyes squinting and her voice slightly shrill, she instructed the students to work for two hours straight in their math books. Two hours straight! So, the four lucky children in the cozy corner in room 6 boldly passed notes and freely giggled between math problems.

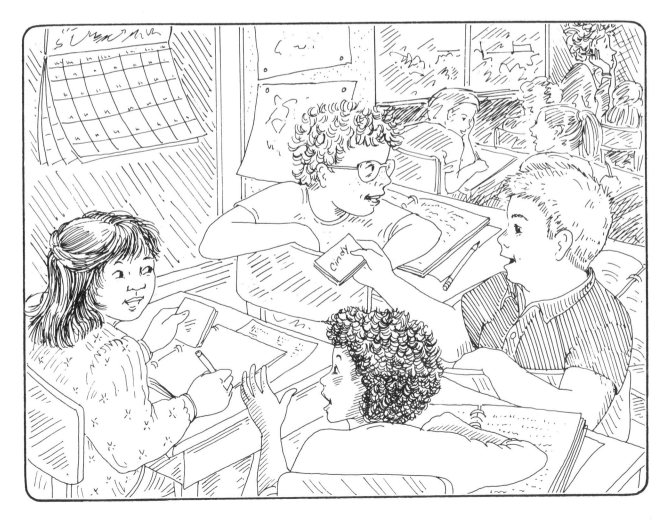

Cindy's desk was at the south side of the cozy corner, right next to the back blackboard. It was so close to the blackboard that when she came home from school most days her grandfather would say, "Now Cindy, your back is so striped with chalk that you look like a very round zebra." At that Grandfather would throw back his head and laugh until his belly shook and tears streamed down the creases in his cheeks.

Cindy would stiffen, plant a scowl on her face, stomp off to the kitchen, flip on the television and plop onto the hard wooden chair next to the cookie jar. Without fail, a round warm voice would softly call out her name again and again. The sound floated up lazily from the cookie jar clown that lived on the counter next to the hard wooden chair.

Being a very obedient girl, Cindy usually answered the round warm voice floating up from the cookie jar clown by reaching up with one hand and gently lifting off the clown's head, careful not to make a single sound. With her other hand, she would reach deep into the clown's tummy to find a bumpy round chocolate chip cookie.

But after school on the day of Ms. Bacon's headache, in March when the fragrance of apple blossoms drifted through the open window, this same round warm voice said something else. As Cindy quietly began to lift off the clown cookie jar's head, it very softly and lovingly said, "Enough is enough," and spun his head around to close the cookie jar tightly.

Cindy jumped back from the chair, her eyes round — as if she'd seen a ghost. It really was the clown cookie jar that spoke. She wasn't imagining it after all. "Enough is enough. Enough is enough? What do you mean?" Cindy muttered, still astonished. The clown hopped down from the counter and tripped over his shoes, turned to face Cindy and smiled broadly.

"Okay, Clown, you are real, but," said Cindy, her eyes narrowing, "where is my cookie? I want my cookie and I want it now!"

"There are no cookies today," replied Clown. "Do you see how empty my suit is? It's just a bag of cloth. I'm too skinny. I'm tired of giving up my cookies to you and only getting skinnier. You're fluffy, soft and round. Could we trade some of your extra fat for some of my extra lean?"

"No way, my friendly clown. I like being round and big. That way if someone doesn't share their lunch with me I can sit on them," Cindy said, and then she blushed.

"Yes, you probably sit on three or four people per day," replied Clown, smirking.

"No, not really. I mean I don't really do that . . . but sometimes I feel like doing that!" continued Cindy.

"That's okay. There are other good reasons to be round. I bet you stay warmer in winter with that extra padding. It must be wonderful to be fluffy, soft and round," sighed Clown.

"Yes, you're right, sort of. But if I think very hard I bet I could find some reasons being round is not very wonderful. For instance, last summer when my mom and I went to visit Aunt Marie in Minneapolis I was sick from the heat. Extra fat makes you feel like you're wearing a fur coat in the middle of a sauna bath."

"You could fan yourself, my sweet Cindy. I'll bet you the top yarn ball from my suit that you can't think of a single way that fat holds you back," said Clown with his round warm voice mixing with the fragrance of the apple blossoms.

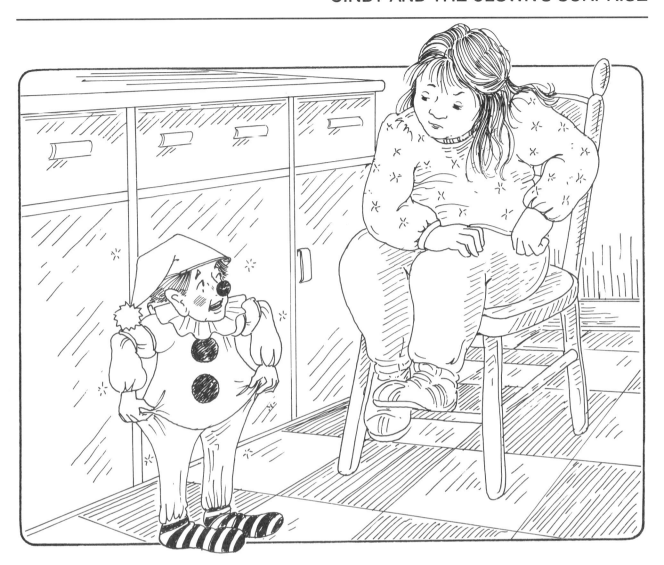

"Yes, I can! Just watch me," said Cindy with a twinkle in her eye. "Of all the kids in the class I can do the least number of sit-ups."

"Nonsense," snorted Clown.

"It's not nonsense! How would you like always being the slowest and being chosen for teams the very, very last every single time?"

"There are worse things, my dear, like forgetting your homework two days in a row or having to clean under your bed," retorted Clown. "I'm not convinced."

"Wait, I have another reason, a good one. All the kids, except of course, my three friends in the cozy corner of room 6, call me names like tub-o

and they snicker and laugh when I go by."

"In my book, Cindy, that's a minor league problem. In fact, it's normal." replied Clown hopping back up onto the counter in case Grandpa came in. "Every single one of the clown cookie jars sitting on the shelf in the Rainbow China Company in Shanghai is teased for something. Some for having their red noses painted on their chins by mistake. Others for having chips of paint gone. And still others for being too tall, too short, too wide, too narrow, too soft, too hard, too cracked or too chipped. Being teased is a fact of life at the Rainbow China Company. Why should it be any different in Ms. Bacon's class?"

Cindy sighed. Would she ever convince

Clown? She scratched her head and her mind wandered to the math problems she had to finish by the next morning. No, she wasn't giving up, "Wait a minute, Clown. I've got a reason!" Cindy said. "Clothes! I can never find great style clothes in my size. How can I take ballet lessons without a leotard that fits?"

Clown reached over to Cindy, putting his arm around her neck and patting her on the shoulder. Then, slowly, Clown shook his head and smiled, "Cindy, your body is round and fluffy. It keeps you warm and makes you feel safe. Anyone can sew stylish clothes in any size at all. They can even sew leotards. It's simple."

"Clown!" said Cindy pulling away, her eyes flashing with anger, "What do you know about being round? It makes me feel safe sometimes, but most times it makes me feel slow and ugly and unlovable. So there!" said Cindy bursting into tears.

Clown looked down at the table. He looked up at the kitchen clock. He gazed at the kitchen counter where the bread crumbs and glob of blueberry jelly still remained from the morning's toast. A big round tear brimmed over his eyelid, rolled down his cheek and dropped onto the kitchen table. It made a bead of wetness on the newly-waxed surface.

Cindy tried to take her mind off feeling wretched and sad. She thought about the glazed, chocolate and white doughnuts with red and green sprinkles on top she had seen on television. She thought about the juicy double cheeseburgers and the crispy fries that left her fingers glistening with grease. And she thought about the round, bumpy chocolate chip cookies in the cookie jar. Suddenly, she wanted one. No, she wanted five. "Oh," said Cindy, astonished, "I know a good thing about being round. You get to eat a lot of cookies. And the cookies block out

my bad feelings. They make me feel better."

Cindy imagined her whole life, day after day, when boredom, sadness or loneliness struck, heading straight for the cookie jar. She thought about not keeping up in P.E. and incessantly thinking about food. She thought of the stomachaches after eating the tenth cookie. It was no fun.

Cindy heard her grandpa shoo the cat off the top of the piano and then bang the screen door on his way out to water the tulips and daffodils in the garden out back. Soon Mom would be home.

At last she crouched down next to the kitchen table so that her dark brown eyes gazed directly into Clown's china blue eyes and said, "I want to lose weight because enough is enough."

The clown quietly nodded. He understood. For a moment the two listened to the sound of the teakettle gently whistling on the stove, ready to make a perfect cup of tea to soothe Grandpa in the late afternoon.

Suddenly the clown's face turned stormy, "Yes, but what about me? I'm skin and bones. I don't think I'll ever get bigger, Cindy. My mother who stores the shortbread biscuits for an English lawyer in Boston and my father who keeps graham crackers for a policeman in Florida are hopelessly skinny. I will be too, no matter what I do."

"Perhaps. You're built like your Mom and Dad. And I'm built like mine. My mom is pretty round and when I went to visit my dad at Christmas, he was more than a little chunky. I figure I'll never look like a broomstick. I'll always be a little bit round—but not as round as I am now. You're built like your skinny parents, so you'll probably always be a little on the scrawny side."

4

Clown thought, shifting his weight from one foot to another, and then sighed. "So I'll always be a little scrawny. Isn't there anything I can do?"

"Sure," replied Cindy, "I just know I can get rid of a lot of my extra fat. If I can get rid of it, well, there's no reason why you can't get more muscle, and a little fat, too. You can get healthy just like I'm going to do. How can you expect to look healthy and grow well on a diet of straight cookies? How can you grow strong muscles when you sit on the counter all day?"

"But Cindy, how will I remember? I'm so busy keeping these cookies fresh and crisp all day that it's easy to forget about eating and exercising."

"I know, Clown. You can set goals each week, like trying to exercise for an hour each day or trying to eat only fruits and veggies for snacks. You can keep track of how many times you really stick with it using STICKER STROKES. I got them this week when I joined SHAPEDOWN. The SHAPEDOWN Club is for kids who are getting in shape. Do you like stickers?

Clown smiled, "You bet, everywhere but on my clown suit. The glue sticks to me and no one bothers to wash it off."

"My mom and grandpa will give me a sticker or some other kind of privilege like watching my favorite television program, helping me with my needle work or, on a weekend day, letting me stay up an hour later every time I make my goals for exercise and food. Plus they are so proud of me. And I'm proud of myself. I've decided to lose six pounds in the next ten weeks, to stop eating sweets when I'm bored or sad and to get in shape by walking, bouncing and dancing. You can do it, too, Clown!

Clown smiled. . . . and winked at Cindy. He could picture himself looking healthier and stronger already. His mother who stores the shortbread biscuits for the English lawyer in Boston and his father who keeps graham crackers for a policeman in Florida had taught him a lot about food and exercise. He just hadn't put all that wisdom into practice—until now! Clown liked the idea of helping Cindy and her friends with SHAPEDOWN while he was getting healthier himself.

With that Clown folded his legs and sat on the counter as still as a cookie jar and Cindy patted him on the cap. Then she ran out the door to plant some carrot seeds in her back garden next to the tulips and the daffodils.

Someone has told you that you are too fat. Maybe they're right, maybe they aren't. What you think is important. This week you will take a good look at your body and decide for yourself if you're too fat.

Even if you are too fat, you may not want to do anything about it right now. Perhaps there are lots of reasons why you don't want to lose weight, like not wanting to cut down on cookies or not wanting to watch less television. On the other hand, there may be reasons why you want to lose weight, like so that the kids will stop teasing you, so that you that can move faster in sports or so that you feel better about yourself.

Think about why you do want to lose weight and why you don't, then decide if you want to lose weight. If you do, SHAPEDOWN. will help you make it happen. Keep in mind that even if your parents want you to lose weight, it will only happen if you make you own decision to lose weight.

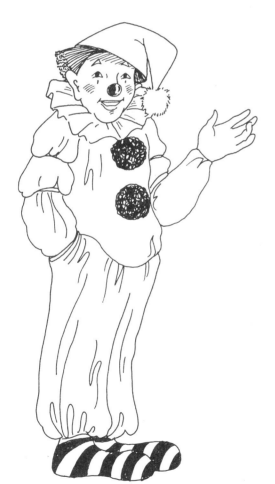

So this week take some time to think about the good and bad things about letting go of extra fat and decide if you want to lose weight.

What is SHAPEDOWN like? There are no shots, pills, fake food, liquid formulas or starvation meal plans. Joining SHAPEDOWN does not mean dieting. Diets don't work. It means each week changing a little bit about your food and a little bit about your exercise. Little changes are things such as having two cookies instead of six, walking a mile to school rather than getting a ride, and eating half a plate of vegetables at dinner. All these little changes add up to a healthy way of living — and to losing weight.

In SHAPEDOWN the whole family joins. You are not alone in making changes. The whole family starts eating lighter — less fatty foods, less sugary foods. The whole family starts moving, too — whether it's on the bike path or on the soccer field. It's not a good idea for you to snack on chips, nor should your skinny brother! Everyone is expected to eat light and exercise, no matter what their weight is.

If you make these changes each week about a pound of extra fat will come off your body each week. That's four cubes of butter off your body per week. Why not more? Because it can hurt your body—by robbing it of muscle rather than fat, decreasing your growth and not giving you enough vitamins and minerals. Plus, to lose more weight per week you have to nearly starve yourself. That makes you grouchy. It makes you feel deprived of food. We do not want you to feel deprived. We want you to enjoy food and your life now more than ever!

YOUR TURN!

Cindy thinks that she is too fat. She has lots of reasons for losing weight and for not losing weight. She has decided she wants to lose weight.

Think about yourself as you answer these questions:

1. Take your clothes off somewhere private and look at your body carefully with a full length mirror. Name three things you like about your body (for example your eyes, your legs, your hands, your ears, your nose or your shoulders):

    1. _____

    2. _____

    3. _____

2. How fat do you think your body is?

    _____ about right

    _____ a little extra fat

    _____ some extra fat

    _____ lots of extra fat

3. The reasons I want to lose weight (check all that are true for you):

    _____ so that I can run and move faster

    _____ so that I'll be better at sports

    _____ so that I can fit into clothes I like

    _____ so that other kids will stop teasing

    _____ so that other kids will like me better

    _____ so that my parents will be even prouder of me

    _____ so that I will be even prouder of myself

    _____ so that _____ .

4. The reasons I do not want to lose weight (check all that are true for you):

_____ because I really like sweets like cookies and candy and don't want to eat fewer of them.

_____ because I really like greasy, fatty foods like chips, butter and cheese and don't want to eat less of them.

_____ because I really like television and don't want limit it to one hour per day.

_____ because I don't want to do more exercise like walking, biking, and playing soccer.

_____ because I am used to my body the way it is and changing it is scary.

_____ because: _____

5. Do you want to lose weight?

_____ yes

_____ no

_____ not sure

6. What are your goals for SHAPEDOWN? What would you like to accomplish in the next 10 weeks?

_____ I want to lose weight: 2   4   6   8   10   pounds

_____ I want to stop gaining weight.

_____ I want to get fit, move better and run faster.

_____ I want to eat regular meals—breakfast, lunch and dinner.

_____ I want to eat less food.

_____ I want to eat fewer sweet foods.

_____ I want to eat fewer fatty, greasy foods.

_____ I want to learn more about food and exercise.

_____ I want to like my body more.

_____ I want to like myself more.

STICKER STROKES

This week you will use your first STICKER STROKES. They help you set goals, get "strokes" of praise, support, rewards, and if you like, stickers. Here's how to use them:

SHAPEDOWN TIME—You and your parent will take five minutes each night to talk about these things:

1. **What went well?** What went well today with your diet and exercise? You will check off all the goals you met.

2. **What did not go well?** You will talk about all the goals you had problems with. You will figure out solutions for next time.

3. **Strokes, praise and rewards!** You will receive rewards for meeting your goals. Also, you and your parent can praise each other for doing such as great job at becoming healthier.

Goals—Each week we'll set some goals that have helped other kids. We think that they will help you, too. Also, you can choose one goal for yourself. It can be anything that helps you eat lighter, exercise more or feel healthier and happier. For instance, you may want to have your bike repaired, buy a bouncer or mini-trampoline, find out about tennis lessons, ask your grandmother to stop offering you cookies and so on.

Strokes—During SHAPEDOWN TIME you can add up how many goals you met. If you met at least five of them in a day, you receive your reward—a pat on the back, a hug from your parent, a sticker, or any other stroke you and your parent agree on. At the end of the week, if you have met at least five of your goals for all seven days, you receive another reward or privilege, like going to a movie, having a friend over, staying up an hour later on a weekend night or renting a favorite videotape, get a pair of earrings, go roller skating or watch MTV for three hours straight.

Weight—Each week you will weigh yourself. Why? Because when you weigh yourself you learn a lot about your habits. You learn whether or not what you are doing is working. If your weight stays the same it means that your exercise and food were just right to keep you even. On the other hand, if your weight goes down about a pound per week, you learn that you are making good changes in your food and exercise.

The scale is not totally accurate. That's because the water, fat, and muscle in your body change day by day. If you drink six glasses of water before you weigh, you'll weigh more! So don't ask yourself how much weight you lose each day. Be more interested in how much you lose over a week or, better yet, a month.

Writing down — Each week you will write down everything you eat for a meal or snack and all of your exercise. For instance, each day this week you will write down your afternoon snacks. Write them down each day before SHAPEDOWN TIME. Write down exactly what you eat and exactly how much you eat. For instance, write down "non-fat milk" rather than "milk" or "whole wheat bread" rather than "bread." To figure out how much you eat use measuring spoons, measuring cups or a food scale. For instance, measure butter in a measuring spoon then scoop it out with a knife and put it on your toast. Pour milk into a measuring cup and then into a glass. Measuring carefully and describing fully the food you eat helps you become more aware of that food you eat and prompts you to eat less and to eat lighter food.

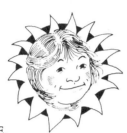

STICKER STROKES

Check if I did it!

Each day I will:

	MON.	TUES.	WED.	THURS.	FRI.	SAT.	SUN.
Take SHAPEDOWN TIME.	X	X	X		X	X	X
Write down what I eat between 2 p.m. and dinner.	X	X	X	X	X	X	X
Eat breakfast, lunch and dinner.	X	X	X	X		X	
Use a healthy family eating style at dinner.	X			X			X
Exercise for 60 minutes or more.	X	X	X	X	X		X
Watch no TV until after I exercise, and limit TV to one hour.	X	X	X	X	X	X	X
My choice: *no cookies*	X	X		X	X	X	X
Number of goals I met:	7	6	5	6	5	5	6

My reward or privilege for making at least five goals every day this week is: *movie with Erin* .

My weight: Start of the week *132* Goal *131* End of the week *130 ½*

STICKER STROKES

Check if I did it!

Each day I will:

Take SHAPEDOWN TIME.

Write down what I eat between 2 p.m. and dinner.

Eat breakfast, lunch and dinner.

Eat only fruits and veggies for snacks.

Exercise for 30 minutes or more.

Watch no TV until after I exercise, and limit TV to one hour.

My choice: _____

Number of goals I met:

My reward or privilege for making at least five goals every day this week is: _____

My weight: Start of the week _____

	MON.	TUES.	WED.	THURS.	FRI.	SAT.	SUN.

___ ___ ___ ___ ___ ___ ___ .

Goal _____   End of the week _____

MY AFTERNOON SNACKS

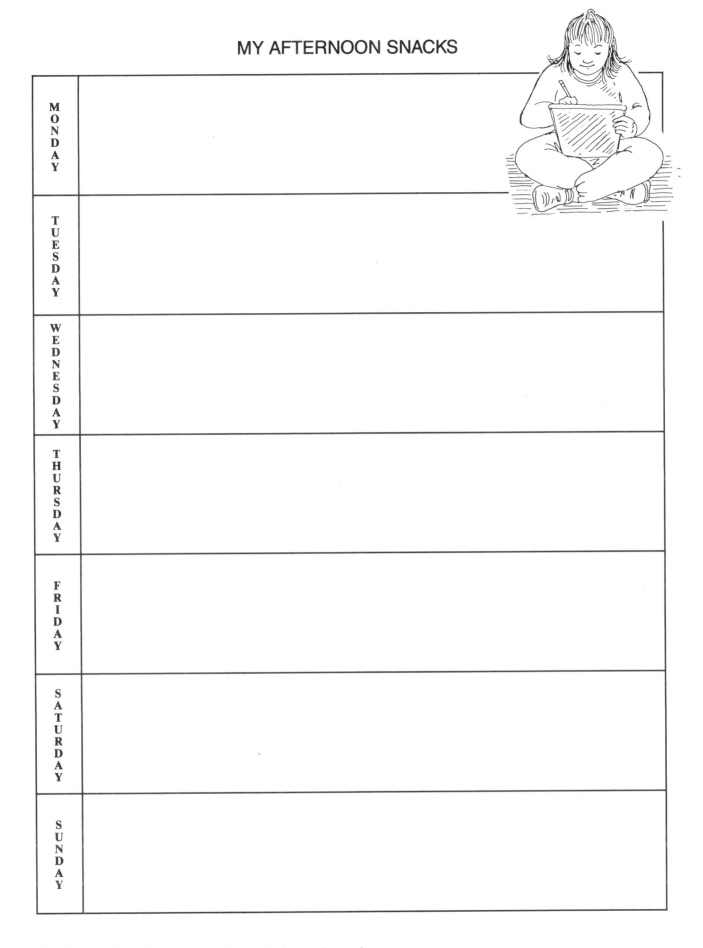

M O N D A Y	
T U E S D A Y	
W E D N E S D A Y	
T H U R S D A Y	
F R I D A Y	
S A T U R D A Y	
S U N D A Y	

Number of days I snacked only on fruits and veggies _____

— JUST FOR FUN! —

PICKING FRUITS AND VEGGIES

You're the boss. Go to the grocery store. You're in charge. Pick out one fruit you love. Pick out a vegetable you like. That's right. What you like matters. Get a veggie and a fruit that please you.

Explore the store.

Don't let anybody interfere. Look at each piece of fruit and each kind of vegetable. Touch it (gently). Smell it. Think about its color, texture and smell.

Pick out one fruit and one vegetable.

Find the exact ones that you think will be flavorful and delicious. Keep them. Pay for them — or ask your parent to pay for them. They're yours.

Eat your fruit and vegetable.

When you eat your fruit and vegetable, describe them. How do they look? How do they feel? How do they taste? Use the words below or make up your own.

fuzzy	waxy	firm	soft	hard	hairy	bumpy	sleek	prickly
seedy	light	heavy	sticky	moist		crunchy	sweet & sour	
pungent	bitter	strong	mellow	creamy	tart	snippy	sharp	

sweet   spicy   tangy   bland   flowery

My fruit
What kind was it?_____

Describe it! _____

My vegetable
What kind was it?_____

Describe it! _____

Talk to your parents. Suggest that each time you go with them to the store that you get your choice of one vegetable and one fruit!

2. MATT AND THE PIZZA PARTY

The very next day at school Ms. Bacon told them that the baby birds were born at the vet's. Her headache had disappeared, too. "Could headaches make baby birds crack their shells and join the world?" asked Ms. Bacon. With the dark circles under her eyes and the furrow in her brow gone, her chocolate brown eyes danced and her mouth curled into a mischievous grin.

The kids in the cozy corner giggled. Cindy chuckled. Amy and Jesse laughed. Matt leaned forward in his chair and pinched Cindy's arm. She turned and playfully slapped his hand.

The kids in the cozy corner were excited because today was their class party. Ms. Bacon's class had sold more pizzas than any other class in the whole school. They had sold pizzas to the postal carriers, fire fighters, and police officers. They had collected pizza orders from their aunts, uncles, cousins, and grandparents. Jesse had even sold a pizza to his neighbor, for his birthday present.

The students in Ms. Bacon's class had sold enough pizza to buy a new backstop for the baseball field. And now their reward — a pizza and ice cream party.

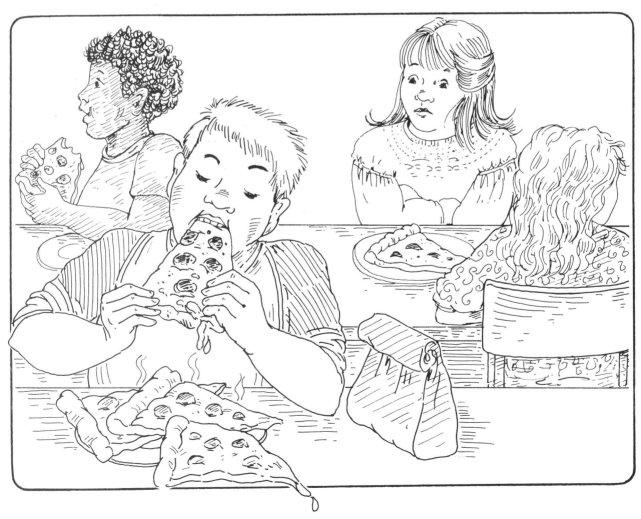

There was only one problem. Ms. Bacon, who frequently forgets announcements when she has headaches, forgot to tell the children about the party. So all of the kids had their regular lunches, too.

Cindy fussed to herself. Eat two lunches? She'd looked over at Matt. He was quiet. Even when he laughed, he laughed very quietly. Matt was a jock, at least he looked like one since he usually wore a football jersey. He was also heavy. Matt was big all over, like Cindy.

Should Cindy ask Matt what to do about lunch? Would he be embarrassed? He had just joined her SHAPEDOWN CLUB, too.

Cindy decided to keep quiet and to watch. She'd watch what Casey did with his lunch. For that matter, she'd keep an eye on Amy and Jesse, too. Neither of them was heavy. Maybe they had the answer.

At that very moment the bell rang so loudly that Cindy jumped. She plugged her ears with her fingers. Matt, Jesse and Amy raced to the door, grabbed their backpacks and raced for the school library. Cindy ran to catch up with them.

In the library on top of the bookshelves were tray upon tray of pepperoni pizza and vegetable pizza, and behind the pizza were 20-gallon containers of rocky road, strawberry and fudge vanilla ice cream, ready for scooping.

Within a split second all of the kids were surrounded by more pizza and ice cream than a person could exercise off in three lifetimes of dancing to MTV, 40 years of running marathons and 800 miles of bike riding.

Just as Cindy was about to eat an entire piece of pepperoni pizza in one very large bite, she stopped, sat back in her chair and played detective. Cindy gazed around the room and caught sight of Jesse and Amy. They each had pieces of vegetable pizza on their paper plates and were slowly munching on them. A scoop of strawberry ice cream was perched on the edge of Amy's plate and a scoop of rocky road on Jesse's. Their lunch bags were half open, with an apple sticking out of Amy's and a green pear on top of Jesse's.

Then she saw Matt. At once her eyes were glued to him. She stared as he stuffed in his mouth bite after bite from one, two, three, four . . . five whole pieces of pepperoni pizza. Around him kids were flying airplanes, jumping up and down and wrestling, but he noticed none of it. All he could think about was getting enough food, eating the pizza and feeling it roll around his tongue and bump its way down his throat.

Suddenly, Matt bounced up from his seat and tore over to where the librarian, Ms. Cakeland, was scooping from 20-gallon containers of rocky road, strawberry and fudge vanilla ice cream. A little river of melted strawberry ice cream ran down her arm and dripped from her elbow. Her hands were caked with sticky ice cream and her hands were ribboned with brown, pink and white goo. In a hushed voice Matt said, "I've been on a diet for two weeks. I'm going to starve right on the spot unless you give me six scoops of ice cream right this minute!" Ms. Cakeland's eyes widened and in an equally hushed voice, she said, "Why of course, Matt, growing boys must eat!" And with that she piled two scoops of rocky road, two of strawberry and two of vanilla fudge onto his plate on top of the crumbs of pizza crust and scraps of pepperoni. Matt smiled and returned to his seat, not knowing that Cindy had watched him each moment.

Cindy pushed away her pepperoni pizza and opened her lunch bag. She brought out her lunch: carrots, celery and broccoli — her ticket to

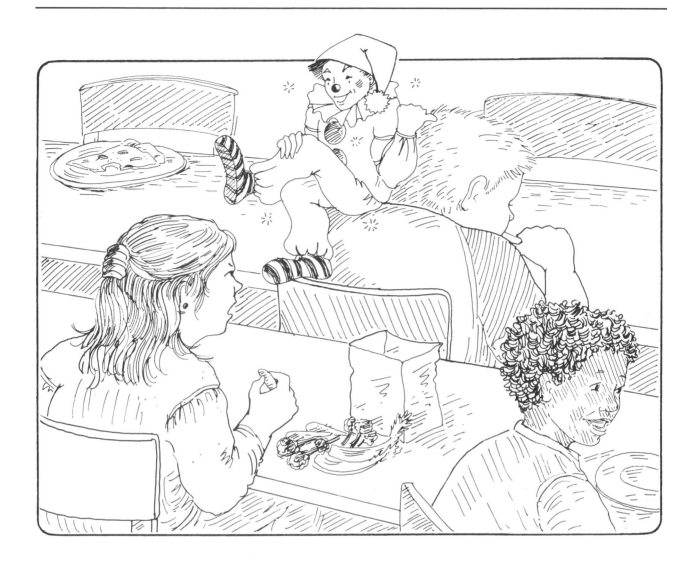

getting lean. Just as she was biting into a very tender carrot, she caught a glimpse of Clown sitting on Matt's shoulder.

Clown leaned back, smiled and said, "Not so smart, my fluffy, soft, round friend. Matt starved himself eating nothing but vegetables for two weeks and look at him now—stuffing himself, chowing down, pigging out, and binge eating. Starving and depriving makes you binge; bingeing makes you fat. Is that what you want for yourself, Cindy, starving and stuffing?

Cindy pulled back from the table and said angrily, "Clown, what are you doing here at school? This is my own turf. Your place is in the kitchen. And besides, Matt will see you!"

Clown just smiled. His face began to fade. His arms and legs and hat faded and only his smile, a very broad, knowing smile remained. In a flash it disappeared, too.

Cindy looked down at her sack full of vegetables. Was she just starving herself? Was she setting herself up to stuff like Matt did?

With that Cindy pushed back her bench, strolled over to the pizza table and snapped up the very last piece of veggie pizza. She sunk her teeth into the crunchy vegetables, gooey cheese and crispy crust. It tasted sooooooo good. She was hungry. The food was light—but not depriving. She was satisfying her hunger and her desire for food. Cindy said "no" to starving—she put away her all veggie lunch. She also said "no" to stuffing—she didn't give a second glance at the pepperoni pizza and ice cream.

Matt leaned back from the table, his stomach hurting. He didn't feel well. The starving hadn't felt good and neither had the stuffing. Maybe his SHAPEDOWN CLUB would help. This sure wasn't working.

Jesse tossed Matt a football. He caught it, almost by reflex, and tucked it under his arm. Matt grabbed his backpack and ran out the door with Jesse in hot pursuit.

SMART TALK

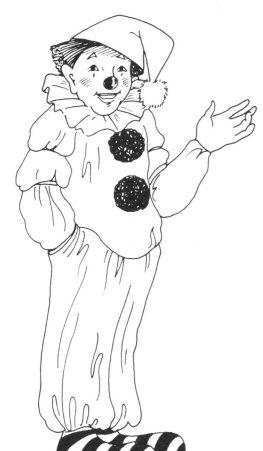

Losing weight doesn't mean dieting. It just means eating healthfully. It means:

Eating regular meals: breakfast, lunch and dinner

Eating more foods low in fat and sugar

Eating small or medium amounts

Let's talk about them one at a time:

Eating regular meals—People who skip meals eat more than people who eat regular meals. If you skip meals you're likely to have lots of snacks. You're apt to snack on foods like chips and cookies. They have more fat and sugar than meals of turkey sandwiches do. Eating regular meals keeps your energy up all day long. A good pattern for most kids is three meals plus an afternoon snack.

Eating more foods low in fat and sugar—No foods are forbidden. All foods, including chips, french fries, candy and cookies are okay some of the time. But you will help yourself lose weight if you eat more lighter foods, foods low in fat and sugar, like an apple rather than apple pie or a baked potato instead of fries.

Eating small to medium amounts—Are cookies really going to make you fatter? No, not if you have one cookie rather than five. Nor will burgers if you have a small one rather than a double

---

SMART TALK continued

cheeseburger. When you really want a sweet or fatty food, have it, but have a small amount.

How do you figure out which foods are lighter and which foods are heavier? We use the SHAPEDOWN Food Summary. It divides food into four groups: FREE FOODS and LIGHT FOODS, which you will eat more often, and HEAVY FOODS and JUNK FOODS which you will eat less often.

FREE FOODS are low in fat and sugar. They get less than 30% of their calories from fat and less than 10% of their calories from sugar. Plus they have so few calories that they don't even count. Enjoy as many FREE FOODS as you like.

LIGHT FOODS are low in fat and sugar just like FREE FOODS. They have more calories than FREE FOODS. You can eat medium amounts of them and still lose weight.

HEAVY FOODS are higher in fat and sugar. Some of them are naturally higher in fat or sugar, like cheese. Others have fat or sugar added to them in processing, like chocolate milk and fries.

JUNK FOODS are mainly fat or sugar. They have many, many calories per bite and almost no vitamins and minerals. Some JUNK FOODS are ready to eat like potato chips. Others you add to other foods, like jam on toast. Eat JUNK FOODS only once in a while, or only in small amounts like a half teaspoon of butter on toast.

Remember, no foods are forbidden. Eat foods from all the groups. But begin to eat FREE FOODS and LIGHT FOODS more often. This week you will pick out foods you want to start eating more of and foods you want to start eating less of. Enjoy experimenting with changing foods!

YOUR TURN!

Cindy and Matt are lightening up their food. They are targeting three FREE FOODS they will eat more often this week. And they are targeting three JUNK FOODS that they will not eat at all this week. Wait a minute. I thought no foods were completely forbidden in SHAPEDOWN. You're right, they are not. But when you want to eat less of a food it helps to quit it completely for a while.

Cindy and Matt chose the foods they want to eat more of and less of this week. Now it's your turn.

1. Please circle all of the FREE FOODS you like. Circle at least ten foods.

FREE FOODS	artichokes	greens	water chestnuts	plain popcorn
	asparagus	jicama	zucchini	tobasco sauce
	bamboo shoots	lettuce	water	soy sauce
	broccoli	mushrooms	mineral water	horseradish
	brussels sprouts	onions	diet soda	garlic
	cabbage	peppers	soda water	onion powder
	carrots	radishes	tea	cinnamon
	cauliflower	sauerkraut	coffee	herbs
	celery	sour pickles	broth	spices
	cucumbers	dill pickles	tomato juice	flavorings
	eggplant	sprouts	vegetable juice	mustard
	green beans	summer squash	limes	vinegar
	green onions	tomatoes	lemons	no-oil salad dressing

2. Circle all of the LIGHT FOODS you like. Circle at least ten of them.

LIGHT FOODS	non-fat milk	fish	papaya	clear soups
	low-fat milk (1%)	tuna, canned	pineapple	vegetable soups
	non-fat buttermilk	in water	peaches	bread
	reduced fat cheese	lean red meat,	plums	bread sticks
	low-fat cottage	all fat removed	raisins	biscuits
	cheese	apples	prunes	english muffins
	plain low-fat	applesauce, canned	strawberries	hamburger buns
	yogurt	without sugar	tangerines	low-fat crackers
	dried beans	apricots	watermelons	unsweetened cereal
	split peas	bananas	fruit, canned	hominy grits
	black-eyed peas	blackberries	in water	tortillas
	lentils	cantaloupe	fruit, canned	plain spaghetti
	refried beans	cherries	in juice	rice cakes
	turkey, light	grapefruit	potatoes	rice
	meat, no skin	grapes	sweet potatoes	bran
	chicken, light	nectarines	peas	barley
	meat, no skin	oranges	winter squash	bulgar

3. Circle all of the HEAVY FOODS you eat often.

HEAVY FOODS	low-fat milk (2%)
	whole milk
	chocolate milk
	cheese
	creamed cottage
	   cheese
	flavored yogurt
	ice milk
	low-fat frozen
	   yogurt
	pudding
	tofu
	peanuts
	peanut butter
		almonds
		sunflower seeds
		chicken or turkey
		   with skin
		chicken or turkey
		   dark meat
		fried chicken
		turkey hot dogs
		fish sticks
		fried fish
		tuna, packed in
		   oil
		red meat
		eggs
			cream soups
			macaroni &
			   cheese
			macaroni salad
			potato salad
			pizza
			chili
			avocado
			sauced vegetables
			fruit rolls
			sweetened
			   applesauce
			fruit, canned
			   in syrup
				coconut
				fries
				hash browns
				sweetened cereals
				granola
				high-fat crackers
				taco shells
				stuffing
				corn bread
				muffins
				pancakes
				waffles
				french toast
				buttered popcorn

4. Circle all of the JUNK FOODS you eat often.

JUNK FOODS	ice cream sherbet shakes cream cheese sour cream half and half whipped cream cream sauce bacon sausage hot dogs salami salt pork	fruit drinks kool-aid jello chips pies cakes cookies doughnuts pastries croissants candy cereal granola candy bars	candy chocolate chocolate topping syrup honey jam jelly marmalade sugar popsicles regular sodas sweet pickles gum	beer wine liquor butter margarine oil lard gravy mayonnaise tartar sauce salad dressing olives salt

5. List three FREE FOODS you will eat more often this week. These are your TARGET FREE FOODS.

_____

_____

6. List three JUNK FOODS you will not eat this week. These are your TARGET JUNK FOODS.

_____

_____

STICKER STROKES

Check if I did it!

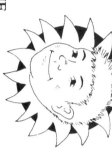

Each day I will:

Take SHAPEDOWN TIME.

Write down what I eat for dinner through bed time.

Eat at least one TARGET FREE FOOD.

Not eat any TARGET JUNK FOODS.

Exercise 45 minutes or more.

Watch no TV until after I exercise, and limit TV to one hour.

My choice: _____

Number of goals I met:

My reward or privilege for making at least five goals every day this week is: _____ .

My weight: Start of the week _____

	MON.	TUES.	WED.	THURS.	FRI.	SAT.	SUN.

— — — — — — —

Start of the week _____   Goal _____   End of the week _____

MY DINNER

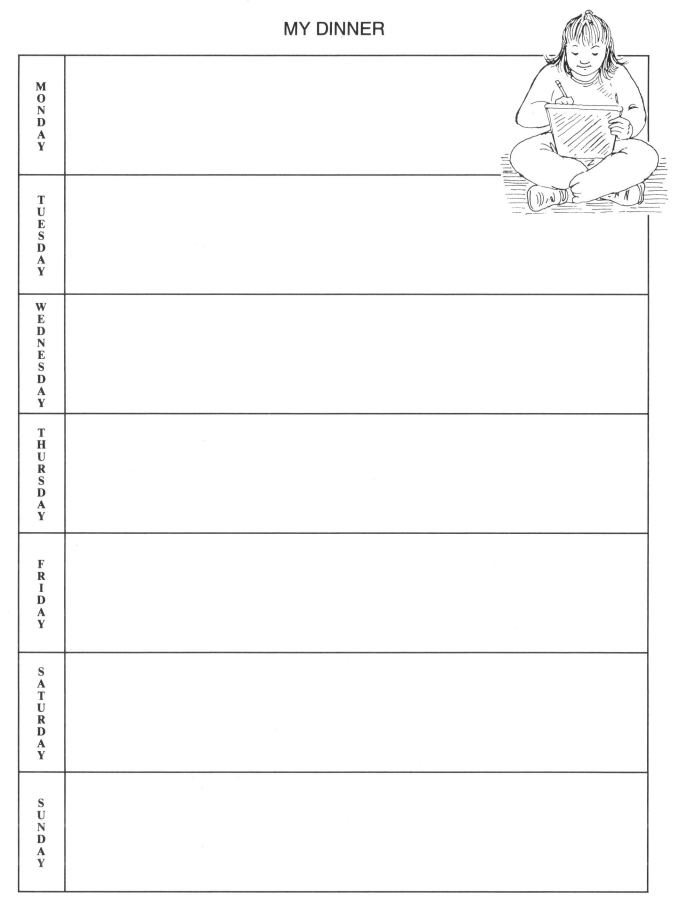

MONDAY	
TUESDAY	
WEDNESDAY	
THURSDAY	
FRIDAY	
SATURDAY	
SUNDAY	

Number of days I ate mainly FREE FOODS and LIGHT FOODS for dinner_____

Number of days I ate foods from all Four Food Groups for dinner_____

JUST FOR FUN!

THROW A POTATO PARTY

Potatoes are light foods. They are rich in complex carbohydrates and don't contain fat. They have vitamins and minerals, too. Enjoy them often!

Are you putting me on?

No way!

Fine, order me up a wheel barrow load of chips, a grocery cart full of fries and a laundry basket full of hash browns.

You're right. There's a catch.

I knew it!

But it's a very small catch. Eat potatoes but don't add fat. That's all there is to it.

When you say fat you mean the baked potato's sour cream blob on top and pool of melted butter underneath? And the lard that they fry potatoes in that makes my fingers slick and greasy? And the puddle of oil they fry the hash browns in that soaks into the potatoes like water soaks into a sponge?

Right. Exactly right!

Oh. So what should I do instead?

Have a potato party. Here's how to do it!

Look for toppings in the grocery store and at home.

Check out the cupboard. Look for herbs and spices that you like. Find sauces that don't have fat in them. At the grocery store find new herb mixtures, spices, seasonings and sauces to try. Here are some toppings that have been kid-tested and rate three star reviews!

lemon juice	sliced green onion	catsup
taco sauce	garlic powder and dill	basil
spaghetti sauce	cottage cheese	chives
Butter Buds	lemon pepper	mint

Bake some potatoes.

Pick out some plump potatoes—one per person. Wash them well. Slit the skin with a sharp knife. Pop them into the microwave or into the oven and cook them until they are soft and fluffy. Cut them into bite-sized pieces—the skin and all. Divide them up, putting them on five small plates. Use a different topping on the potato bites on each plate.

Enjoy your potato tasting!

Bite into each piece and taste it. How did it taste? Rate them each below.

Topping I tried	How I liked it				
	bad		OK		good
_____	1	2	3	4	5
_____	1	2	3	4	5
_____	1	2	3	4	5
_____	1	2	3	4	5
_____	1	2	3	4	5

3. MATT AND CINDY'S PRIVATE CLUB

Matt sat in the cozy corner of Ms. Bacon's room the day after the pizza and ice cream party with his stomach still hurting from the five pieces of pepperoni pizza and the six scoops of rocky road, strawberry and fudge vanilla ice cream.

He was writing the next sentence in his composition, "My Experience with an Unidentified Flying Object," about his plane trip to Disney World, when his pencil broke. He got up, squeezed past Cindy and strode straight to the pencil sharpener. He heard a "wapppp" and felt a sharp bump on his back. Somebody in the

front row, probably David, had hit him with a spit wad.

There was a hush. Then a giggle. Matt's face turned as red as a pomegranate. They were giggling about his weight! They were laughing at him! Matt prayed that he would melt into the floor, turn into dust and blow away so that he would never have to turn around and face them all.

Matt pulled in his swollen stomach, took a deep breath, turned on his heels and walked

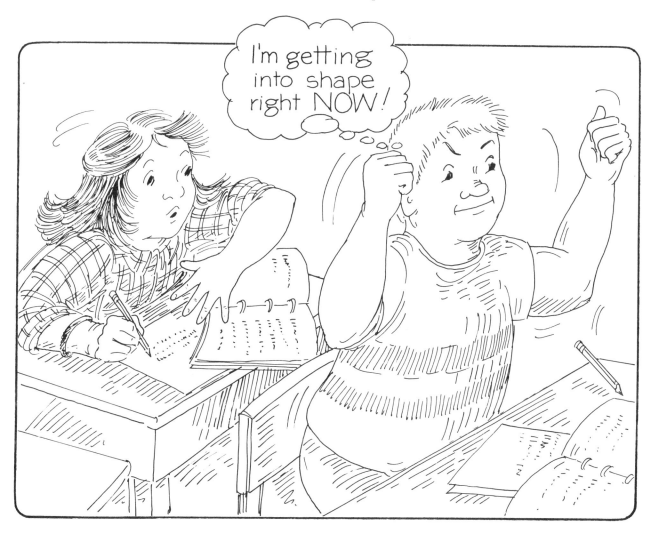

slowly back to his seat with his head held high. The class quietly went back to writing their compositions. They were quiet, that is, until Amy went up to ask Ms. Baker how to spell the capital of Nebraska, which is where she went during spring break. Then they started snickering about Amy's skinny arms.

Back in his seat, Matt lowered his head, curled his body over his desk and placed his pencil to his paper to write out the next sentence—the one that told about the flashing lights—when snap! His pencil broke again. He heard it snap, he saw the little black cone-shaped tip roll down his desk, but he didn't believe it. How could it break again?

Was life always going to be so difficult? Was he doomed to be fat because his mother was chunky and because his dad was so big? Was it written in his genes that he'd be fat forever? When would the teasing and tormenting stop?

Just then Cindy tapped him on the shoulder. He looked up to see her smiling face. She handed him a freshly sharpened pencil.

He looked over and gave her a half smile. Cindy had saved him.

Matt thought again about his family. The night before, he had watched his mother, father and sister Kate, closely. They all had eaten greasy, fatty, sugary foods. Last night his sister had eaten six chocolate chip cookies and his father seven! All they ever did was eat and watch television.

Matt's brow furrowed. Did he want a fat life or a thin life? Was eating light and exercising worth it? Yes, thought Matt, I'm not waiting around any more. I'm getting in shape right now! As he said "Now" Matt jumped in his chair. Cindy jumped, too and then they both laughed.

Cindy passed Matt a note:

"I think you're cute." All around the border of the white paper were pink hearts.

Matt read it, and wrote back:

"I'm glad we're starting SHAPEDOWN together."

Cindy blushed.

Matt wondered what would happen to his family if he started eating light, exercising and losing weight. Would they be mad at him? Would they feel that he was showing them up? Would they feel proud of him? Matt thought as he added the last sentence to his composition. "The flashing white lights were gone for now, but would they return? Perhaps, tonight!" He underlined "Perhaps, tonight!" five times and turned over his paper.

No, they wouldn't be mad at him for getting in shape. They'd be proud. Besides Matt would help them, too. Maybe Matt's weight would be a way to get his mom and dad in shape. Matt could help the whole family!

After Ms. Baker gave them their science homework assignment, Matt picked up his books and was ready to charge out the door. He stopped. Matt turned to Cindy, "Wanna ride bikes to school together tomorrow?"

Cindy nodded, "Sure, see you tomorrow at seven-thirty in front of my house," and ran out the door.

That night Cindy sat at the kitchen table and thought about Matt and bike riding. Just then Clown, now stuffed with rice crackers, hopped down from his shelf and walked across the table.

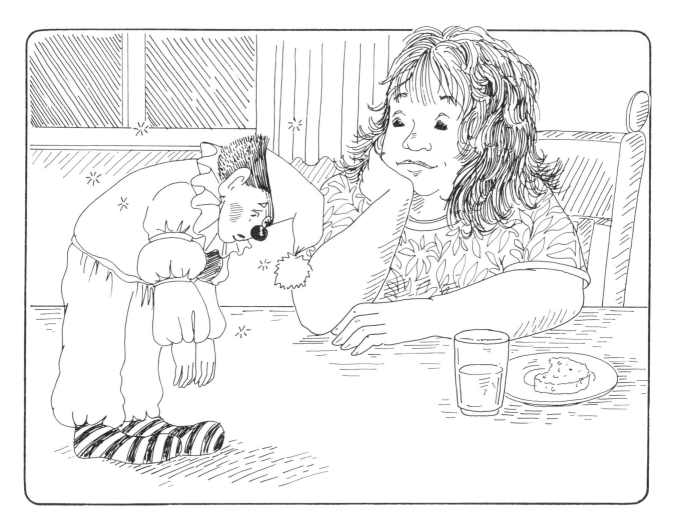

"Cindy," said Clown, "Have you noticed that I've filled out?"

"Yes, Clown," said Cindy affectionately, "Those rice crackers really filled you out without making you too fat."

"But Cindy," continued Clown, "Just look at my arms. Can you see any muscles?"

Cindy opened her eyes very wide and then shook her head, "Not one, Clown."

"I haven't an ounce of strength, Cindy. I can't even climb up to the top shelf to change my cookies . . . or crackers, that is. And watch this," he said bending over, "I can't even touch my knees, let alone my toes."

"Well, you're not the most flexible clown in the universe, Clown, but you're still the best cracker jar I've ever known." said Cindy standing up and bending down to touch her toes . . . and only reaching her knees.

"What's worse," said Clown, "is that I can't even walk up the hill to my cousin Owl's, who was stuffed with oatmeal raisin cookies last week. Who knows what's filling him up this week!"

"Clown, you don't have much endurance, do you? That's no fun! I'll help you, Clown. My friend, Matt and I have a SHAPEDOWN CLUB. We're getting in shape. We're starting tomorrow to do BODY STRETCHES for flexibility, BODY BUILDERS for strength and

HUFF AND PUFF exercises for endurance. We're going to get so fit that we can have fun for hours and hours without getting tired!"

"And I will be able to walk up the hill to see what kind of cookies my Cousin Owl's stuffed with, and touch my toes and climb up to the highest shelf?"

"You bet, Clown, if you exercise almost every day for an hour or more," said Cindy with a wink, and lifted Clown's hat to help herself to a cracker. "Matt and I are starting tomorrow. We're biking half an hour to school and half an hour back! That's a HUFF AND PUFF exercise."

Clown took off his hat and scratched his head. "OK, you're doing the biking to make your heart and lungs strong and to give you endurance. But what are you doing to be flexible and strong?" he questioned.

Cindy smiled, "When I get up in the morning I'm going to do BODY STRETCHES and for my BODY BUILDERS I'm going to dig in Grandpa's garden for strength.

"I wish I had a plan," said CLOWN sadly.

"You can, Clown. Just imagine ways to move your body that are fun!"

"Oh!" said Clown, "I know! For HUFF AND PUFFS, I'll walk up the hill to Cousin Owl's twice a day."

"Great. That will get your heart and lungs strong. Then you can run and play without getting tired!" replied Cindy.

Clown jumped down onto the table. "For my BODY STRETCHES, I'll touch my toes 20 times in the morning and 20 times at night. For BODY BUILDERS I'll lift all of the canned peaches, pears and plums from the bottom shelf to the top shelf and back before lunch and before dinner."

Clown leaned back and smiled. He had made his own exercise plan!

Just after dawn the next morning Cindy rolled out of bed and looked at her body in the mirror. It looked fluffy and round. She had a very comfortable body. The fat felt like it was hugging her. There were good things about letting go of extra fat, but she would probably miss the coziness of her round body.

Cindy started her morning BODY STRETCHES, stretching way up high, over to one side and then like a swing, over to the other. She imagined herself looking leaner. She pushed in her cheeks looking for her cheekbones. She felt her legs looking for muscles. If she got leaner she would still be Cindy, but just a leaner, fitter Cindy. Maybe being a leaner, fitter Cindy would be pretty cozy, after all.

The stretching felt good. With her clothes on, teeth brushed, hair combed, books in hand, Cindy ran down the stairs, spooned a bowl of wheat flakes — real cereal, not the candy-coated kind — and non-fat milk into her hungry body and raced out the door, just in time to see Matt bike up her street.

─ **SMART TALK** ─

Why am I heavy?—You are not to blame for being heavy. It is not your fault. There are lots of reasons people are heavy. Most times there are several reasons. The most common reasons are:

Fat genes   inheriting a body from your parent that tends to be round

Being sick   not being able to exercise because of asthma or always getting colds, or taking medicines that put on weight

Food   eating too much
not eating regular meals (breakfast, lunch, dinner)
eating too much fat and sugar

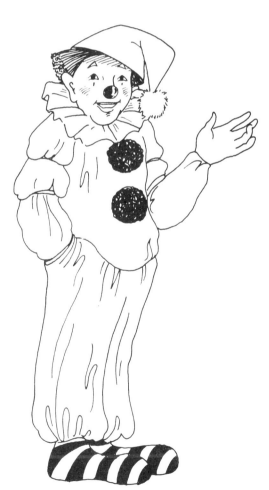

Activity   sitting down rather than exercising an hour or so a day
keeping busy by eating rather than by doing fun, helpful or interesting things
watching more than one hour of television per day

Feelings   feeling sad, lonely, bored, or unloved
not liking yourself or your body
feeling worried or anxious

Knowledge   not knowing how to eat and exercise to get leaner

Family   parent or family having troubles
parents having a hard time saying "no" to you and making it stick
parents not knowing how to help you feel loved, valued and reassured
family eating a lot, not eating regular meals, eating too much fat or sugar
family not exercising or getting its fun from food not activities

---

SMART TALK continued

Other kids	being with friends who eat a lot of JUNK FOOD
	having other kids offer you JUNK FOOD
	being teased by other kids about weight
School	having school problems
	having food at school that is mainly HEAVY FOOD and JUNK FOOD
Other	many other things like going to a church that gives you JUNK FOOD
	or watching TV JUNK FOOD commercials

Often these reasons are like dominoes lined up. When one falls it knocks over the next one. For instance, Jason's parents were fighting. That made Jason worried. To block out the feelings of worry he ate more. When he ate more he gained weight and didn't feel like exercising, so he watched more television. Soon he was in the habit of eating chips, watching television and not seeing his friends after school. That just made him gain more weight. So Jason's dominoes that led to his gaining weight were: parent's troubles, feeling worried, eating high fat foods, watching television, not exercising, stopping seeing friends.

Think about the dominoes that help put weight on you! Figuring out your own dominoes makes it easier to lose weight. You know what has caused your weight. Everything — except fat genes — can often be changed. Even fat genes really don't make you heavy. They make the difference between being slightly rounded and looking like a broomstick, that's all.

Exercise is part of SHAPEDOWN because it's fun and because it makes you healthier. It also helps you lose weight, feel less hungry and changes you body from fat to lean. It gives you a "glow" and shrinks your troubles down to size. It makes you enjoy your body more.

How long do I exercise? You can quickly work up to 60 minutes per day. Start with 30. Go to 45 and then finally 60. Recess and P.E. class at school don't count. You're already doing them and still have a weight problem. That means you need more exercise.

How often do I exercise? Every day. Your body needs food every day. Your body also needs exercise every day. Otherwise the poor little blood vessels shrink, your energy-boosting enzymes go away and your body feels restless and couped up. Give your body the exercise it needs to stay pleased as punch every day.

When do I exercise? Any time is a good time, but make it a regular time — like every morning after breakfast or every night after dinner. For most kids the best time is immediately after school. That's because right then they are tired or hungry and exercise takes away that hunger and tiredness. Exercise is a great break before starting your homework.

What kind of exercise? Any kind of exercise that is safe and doesn't hurt your body when you do it is good. Standing is better than sitting. Walking is better than standing. The idea is to move.

There are three parts to fitness: strength, flexibility and endurance. You needs all three kinds of fitness to make your body work at its best.

Strength is how strong you are — for instance, how much weight your muscles can lift. Most exercise makes you stronger. Chores like stacking firewood or carrying in groceries strengthen your muscles and so do floor exercises. For instance, doing sit-ups strengthens your stomach muscles. It doesn't take the fat off your stomach, but it does strengthen the muscles underneath. Activities that makes your muscles stronger we call BODY BUILDERS.

Can you make yourself look like a pretzel? If you can, you're very, very flexible! Being flexible means you can touch your toes without a bit of strain. Activities that make your body bendable and flexible we call BODY STRETCHES. By stretching your body you teach it a lesson in acting like a pretzel.

Most kids want to run fast and be good at sports. Sure, you need to be strong and flexible for most sports, too, but mainly you need to have energy. Your body can't poop out on you half way through a game. You need to have good endurance. How do you make your heart and lungs strong so you can run and play without getting tired? With HUFF AND PUFF exercises. They are also the ones that burn up fat.

Don't go too fast. Is sprinting a good HUFF AND PUFF exercise? No! People who sprint and exercise too fast just tire themselves out and — worse — get themselves injured. Exercise in which you breathe hard (but not too hard!) like brisk walking, biking, and bouncing on the mini-trampoline burns up fat, boosts your endurance and makes your heart and lungs strong.

To be sure you are not underexercising or overexercising, take your pulse right after exercising. If for 6 seconds it is 12 to 15 beats, your exercise is just right. If it's more than 15, slow down. If it's less that 12, speed up.

How do I get ready to be lean? People have told you you should lose weight. You think that you should lose weight. But you might not be comfortable weighing less. It may feel strange. You look at your body and it doesn't look like your own. What happened to your cheeks and your stomach? They seemed to disappear.

SMART TALK continued

People act differently toward you. They don't tease you as much. But also, your friends change. Maybe some of your friends will stop liking you and others will start liking you. To make yourself more comfortable with the lean body you're creating, picture yourself thinner. How does it feel? How do your look? Picture it often so that as you lose extra fat, your new lean body will seem normal.

YOUR TURN!

Matt thought about the dominoes that helped him gain extra fat. Think about what you think are your very own dominoes.

1. I think that the things that helped me gain extra fat are (check all that apply to you):

_____ fat genes

_____ being sick

_____ eating too much

_____ not eating regular meals

_____ not enough exercise

_____ bored, not busy enough

_____ watching more than one hour of television per day

_____ feeling sad, lonely, bored or unloved

_____ not liking myself

_____ not liking my body

_____ feeling anxious or worried

_____ not knowing how to eat and exercise to lose weight

_____ parent or family having troubles

_____ parents have a hard time saying "no" and making it stick

_____ parents not knowing how to help me feel loved and secure

_____ family eating a lot

_____ family not eating regular meals

_____ family eating foods high in fat or sugar

_____ family not exercising much

_____ family getting its fun from food not from activities

_____ friends offering me JUNK FOODS

_____ other kids teasing me about weight

_____ having school problems

_____ food at school being high in fat or sugar

_____ other:_____

2. Matt made up his exercise program: Stretching for 5 minutes every morning before breakfast and right before soccer for BODY STRETCHES, 30 sit-ups and 15 push-ups every night for BODY BUILDERS, and an hour of biking, soccer or the bouncer (mini-trampoline) for HUFF AND PUFF exercises. What is your plan?

BODY STRETCHES
What I will do: _____

BODY BUILDERS
What I will do: _____

HUFF AND PUFF
What I will do: _____

_____

_____

When I will exercise on week days: (Circle all that apply to you):

before school   after school   before dinner   after dinner

When I will exercise on weekends (Cricle all that apply to you):

morning   afternoon   evening

Who I will exercise with (Circle all that apply to you):

mother   father   sister   brother   friend

neighbor   whole family   other _____

3. Cindy rested on her bed quietly. She closed her eyes and relaxed. She pictured herself becoming leaner and leaner. Her cheekbones began to show. He face was longer and her eyes and nose looked bigger. Her arms and stomach were smaller. She felt light. It felt strange. She looked different. It felt good, mostly.

Picture yourself leaner. Describe how your face and body look different:

_____

_____

How did it feel to be leaner? (check all that are true for you):

_____ great

_____ OK

_____ scary

_____ uncomfortable

_____ impossible

_____ bad

_____ other_____

STICKER STROKES

Check if I did it!

	MON.	TUES.	WED.	THURS.	FRI.	SAT.	SUN.

Each day I will:

Take SHAPEDOWN TIME.

Write down my exercise.

Do chores for 30 minutes or more.

Do enriching activities for 30 minutes or more.

Exercise for 60 minutes or more.

Watch no TV until I exercise, and limit TV to one hour.

My choice: _____

Number of goals I met: ____ ____ ____ ____ ____ ____ ____

My reward or privilege for making at least five goals every day this week is: _____.

My weight: _____ Start of the week _____ Goal _____ End of the week _____

37

Kids ON THE MOVE!

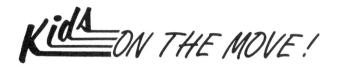

	MINUTES	ACTIVITY
MONDAY		
TUESDAY		
WEDNESDAY		
THURSDAY		
FRIDAY		
SATURDAY		
SUNDAY		

---JUST FOR FUN!---

Circle the names of vegetables in the puzzle below. Can you find all twelve? (Two are on the diagonal.)

```
S  L  E  T  T  U  C  E  O
J  S  A  P  C  C  O  R  T
I  P  K  A  A  E  L  O  P
C  I  H  R  B  L  L  M  O
A  N  L  S  B  E  A  A  T
M  A  B  L  A  R  R  I  A
A  C  S  E  G  Y  D  N  T
D  H  P  Y  E  F  I  E  O
E  T  O  M  A  T  O  S  H
```

Which of the vegetables you circled are not leaves? Please list them:

_____

_____

Name one of these vegetables that you will eat this week:

_____

Did you eat it?   YES   NO

Describe how it looked, tasted and felt:_____

_____

_____

4. TRADING LUNCHES

Matt watched Cindy run out of her house, grab her bike and pedal down her driveway toward him. Cindy looked pretty and vibrant today. She carried her books under her arm . . . but where was her lunch? For that matter, where was Matt's lunch?

"Lunch," said Matt. "Lunch."

"Oh, I forgot!" exclaimed Cindy.

"We both forgot."

"Let's just buy it at school, Matt," suggested Cindy, "it's so easy."

"Cindy, people in our SHAPEDOWN CLUB think that greasy stuff at school is gross!"

"Oh!" said Cindy, throwing her head back and rolling her eyes. "They're right. It is gross. You can just see the grease and fat oozing out of the fries and dripping off the burritos. Yuck!"

"And crusted sugar flaking off the doughnuts. Sticky sugar in candy ready to breed bugs on your teeth. Gross!" added Matt.

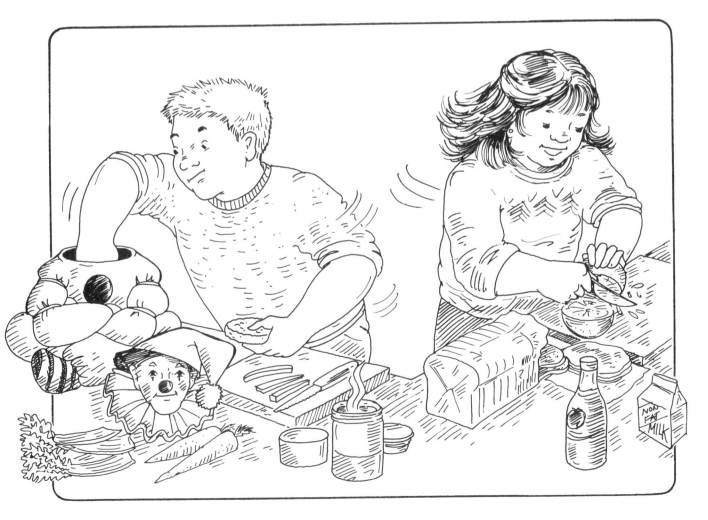

41

"We could go to the market down the street, the one with the video games," suggested Cindy.

"The only choices they have are sodas, candy and all that fat food you pop into the microwave. There isn't a real piece of food in the place!" cracked Matt.

"I know!" said Cindy, "Let's go to my house and fix our own lunches."

With that, the two members of the SHAPE-DOWN CLUB ran through the back screen door and into the kitchen. They could hear Cindy's mother and grandfather upstairs getting ready for the day.

Matt opened the refrigerator and saw a big yellow bowl of veggies, crisp, fresh and ready-to-eat. "There's our lunch right there," said Matt with a noble nod.

"Matt, lunch shouldn't just be veggies. People lose extra fat all the time by eating regular food, not just celery sticks. Straight veggies will just make you feel hungry and deprived and then you'll just, you'll just . . . ."

"I know. Binge. Right?" said Matt looking rather sheepish.

"Yes, you're right. Food is something to eat when you're hungry. It's not something to feel guilty about or afraid of. Let's make a lunch that's light but that will take away our hunger and taste good!

"I know how to load up on hamburgers, fries, sodas, chips and cookies, and I know how to starve myself. I guess I haven't learned yet how to eat!"

"Simple. Just eat lots of different kinds of

LIGHT FOODS and FREE FOODS. Let's make a lunch for each other and trade. We'll both be surprised at lunch time!"

Matt and Cindy raced around the kitchen, peeking in the cupboard, refrigerator, and even inside Clown. They each chopped, stirred, spread, sliced and bagged a lunch. Suddenly, they heard Grandpa's steps on the stairs. In a wink, Matt and Cindy, bag lunches in hand, quietly slipped out the back screen door, ran for their bikes and were off to school.

The wind whistled by their ears, leaves danced around their wheels and the morning air froze their noses and reddened their cheeks. Up the hills they huffed and puffed. Down the slopes they soared, and finally landed at school. Giggling and shouting they tossed the lunches to each other. Each then held a surprise bag.

By lunch time Matt just knew he'd guessed everything in the lunch, just from feeling the bag. Cindy's bag felt like it had a round hard lump in it and a few soft, squishy things. The lunch bell ran and they were off to the lunch area. But Amy stopped them, "Want a cherry fruit roll? I've got an extra!"

Cindy looked at Matt. She didn't want Amy to know she was trying to lose weight. Matt quickly whispered in her ear, "Just say, 'No thanks.'"

Cindy said, "No thanks, Amy." Amy looked quizical. Everybody loves fruit rolls. Oh well, thought Amy, I'll just ask someone else.

"But Matt," protested Cindy, "shouldn't I give her a reason? What will she think?"

"You could say, 'No thanks, I'm not hungry.' or 'No, thanks, I have enough lunch.' But all you

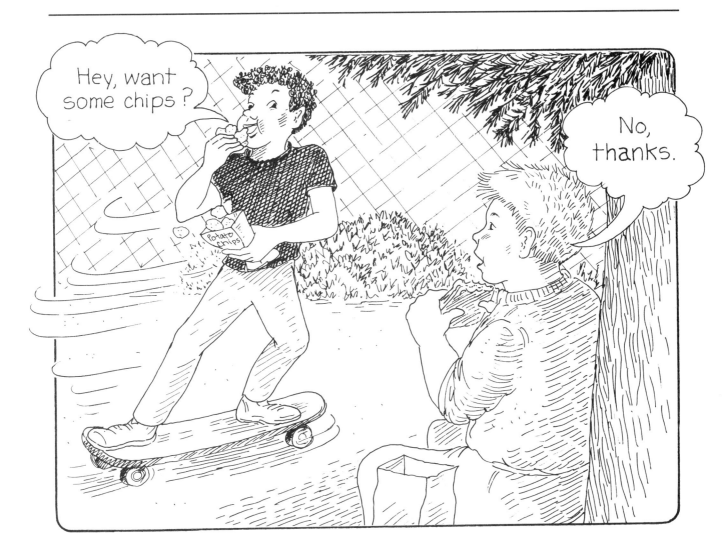

really need to do is say 'No thanks.' What she thinks is not as important as what you think. You need to take care of yourself, not to worry about what everyone thinks. Besides, if she stops being your friend because you didn't eat her fruit roll, she wasn't much of a friend anyway."

Cindy listened and knew Matt was right. She liked their club. They were really helping each other.

Cindy and Matt found a place to eat on a bench under a large pine tree and hurriedly tore open their bags.

Matt discovered a turkey sandwich on whole wheat with—not mayonnaise—but ketchup. A big, sweet orange sliced up and a small carton of non-fat milk. He was hungry and bit right into his sandwich.

Just then David sailed by on his skateboard—which is not allowed in the lunch area. "Hey, Matt, want some chips?" he said, stuffing a handful into his mouth.

"No thanks," said Matt.

Cindy tore open her bag. In it was her old red thermos filled with vegetable soup, a baggie of carrot sticks and another baggie of celery. And two crackers from Clown's tummy. Cindy laughed. Three servings of veggies and one of grains. That's progress, Matt!" and she laughed as she munched on a sweet, crisp carrot stick.

43

SMART TALK

Eating—Your parents will tell you when it's time to eat and the foods you can have. You will decide whether you eat and how much you eat.

It is your parent's job to be in charge of the times and kinds of food you eat. You control whether or not you eat and how much you eat. That is your job. Nothing goes into your mouth that you don't put there.

How do you decide how much to eat? If the food is a HEAVY FOOD or a JUNK FOOD you eat very little of it. If it's a FREE FOOD or a LIGHT FOOD you eat more of it. You also decide based on your hunger. If you've been eating way more than your body needs, your body can fool you. You have trained your body to want more food. If you start exercising and eating less, soon your body will get back to normal. Then it will give you some idea of how much food you need.

Eat a little more when you feel hungry and a little less when you don't feel as hungry. Eat until your are just satisfied, not stuffed. Look at the HUNGER SCALE below. When you feel the hunger vanish, stop right then. Push away your plate when you are just satisfied. You are done.

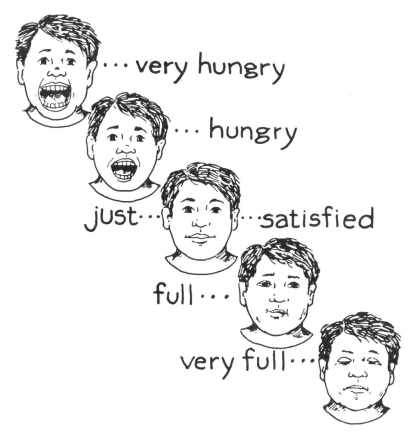

···very hungry

··· hungry

just··· ···satisfied

full ···

very full···

Fixing lunch — Lots of kids fix their lunches on school days, for picnics or for weekend lunches. What's a healthy bag lunch? A basic healthy lunch is:

a whole or half sandwich

a piece or two of fruit

a baggie full of veggies

non-fat milk

water

Pack as many veggies as you like. Use whole wheat or other whole grain bread because it gives you a whole wallop more nutrition than white bread does.

Pay attention to whether you have fatty foods in your sandwich. Bread is a LIGHT FOOD, but most of the things you put between bread are heavy. Steer clear of more than a smidgen of mayonnaise, and stick to turkey and other low fat meats rather than greasy fillings like salami and oil-packed tuna. Why? Because fat goes to fat. Fat has more than twice the calories of carbohydrates and proteins.

Speaking up — Sometimes people will offer you food when your parents aren't around. Kids at school will offer you chips and granola bars. Grandmothers and neighbors will push cookies on you. You can take these foods every time your parent isn't looking. But that won't make you feel good. You'll feel like you did something you weren't proud of. You'll weigh yourself each week and find that you haven't lost weight.

Remember that eating is a private and personal choice. It is your choice. Only you put food in your mouth. Nobody else puts it there but you. When you're on your own — at a friend's or at school — you will make choices for yourself. Don't eat just because someone offers you food. You are not a little child. You are almost a teenager and you are more responsible than a little child is. You can make choices you are proud of.

When someone offers you food, think about three things:

1. Is it time to eat (breakfast, lunch, snack or dinner)?

If it isn't, don't eat.

SMART TALK continued

2. Is the food a LIGHT FOOD or FREE FOOD?

If it isn't, **don't eat it.** Eat your meal or snack later. Or **do eat it** but eat only half of it.

3. Am I hungry?

If you aren't hungry, eat little or none of it. Wait until your next meal or snack to eat.

When you decide not to eat something someone offers you, tell them directly. Just say "No thanks!," "No, thanks I'm not hungry." or "No thanks, I don't feel like cookies right now." Speak up politely and directly and say, "No, thanks!"

YOUR TURN!

1. Matt practiced listening to his hunger signals. He practiced stopping eating when he was just satisfied. He tried to stop before he was full or very full. Use the hunger scale each time you eat this week to figure your hunger when you stopped eating. Circle how you felt after three meals or snacks of your choice.

Day	Meal	How I felt when I stopped eating:
_____	breakfast lunch snack dinner	very hungry hungry just satisfied full very full
_____	breakfast lunch snack dinner	very hungry hungry just satisfied full very full
_____	breakfast lunch snack dinner	very hungry hungry just satisfied full very full

YOUR TURN!

2. Look at your FOOD SUMMARY at the back of this book. Find the FREE FOODS and LIGHT FOODS you enjoy. Fill up your lunch bags below with two lunches that are light and taste good.

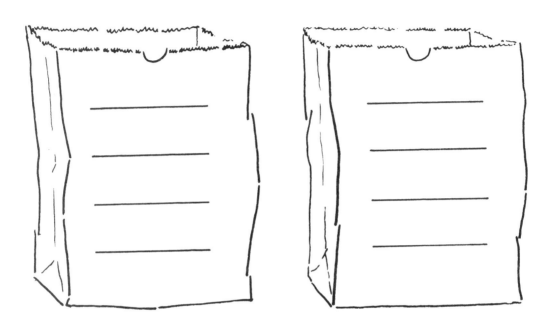

3. Look at the FOOD SUMMARY at the back of this book. List three LIGHT FOODS you will eat more often this week. These are your TARGET LIGHT FOODS.

_____

_____

_____

4. List three HEAVY FOODS you will not eat this week. These are your TARGET HEAVY FOODS.

_____

_____

_____

5. Think about the three questions to ask yourself when someone offers you food. Remember the three questions:

    1. Is it time to eat (breakfast, lunch, snack or dinner)?

    2. Is the food a LIGHT FOOD or FREE FOOD?

    3. Am I hungry?

Describe one time this week when you asked yourself these three questions.

_____

_____

_____

6. If you decided that you did not want the food someone offered you what would you say?

To a friend who offers you a cookie:

_____

To your mother or father who offers you a bag of chips (even parents sometimes offer you food that isn't good for you).

_____

To a grandmother or older friend who wants to buy you a candy bar?

_____

STICKER STROKES

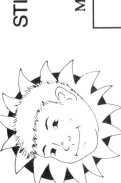

Check if I did it!

	MON.	TUES.	WED.	THURS.	FRI.	SAT.	SUN.
Each day I will:							
Take SHAPEDOWN TIME.							
Write down what I eat for lunch.							
Eat at least one TARGET LIGHT FOOD.							
Not eat any TARGET HEAVY FOODS.							
Exercise for 60 minutes or more.							
Watch no TV until after I exercise, and limit TV to one hour.							
My choice: _____							

Number of goals I met: ____ ____ ____ ____ ____ ____ ____

My reward or privilege for making at least five goals every day this week is: _____ .

My weight: _____ Start of the week _____ Goal _____ End of the week _____

49

MY LUNCH

MONDAY	
TUESDAY	
WEDNESDAY	
THURSDAY	
FRIDAY	
SATURDAY	
SUNDAY	

Number of days I ate mainly FREE FOODS and LIGHT FOODS_____

Number of days I ate foods from all Four Food Groups for lunch_____

---JUST FOR FUN!---

BE A FAT FINDER

There it is lurking in your tuna sandwich, hiding in your chicken drumstick and slipping over your lettuce leaves and around your tomato slices in your salad. What is it? FAT. The three letter word — FAT.

Explore the store

Be a fat finder this week. Get the facts from your grocery store. Seek them out and track them down. Be equipped with the facts about fat.

The ground rules

Use labels as your guide. Key in on two facts: calories per serving and grams of fat per serving. With these facts you can uncover the truth about a food. You can tell in a minute if it's mainly fat.

The formula

Each gram of fat has 9 calories. The label tells you how many total calories in a serving and how many grams of fat in a serving. So use this formula:

$$\frac{\text{Grams of fat X 9}}{\text{Calories}}$$

The answer

If the formula tells you that it's more than 30, it's a heavier food. If it's 30 or less, its a lighter food.

Now, turn the page and become a fat finder.

JUST FOR FUN!

Go to the store and find the grams of fat and calories per serving of these foods, plus three others that you choose. When you come home use the formula to figure out how much fat each food has. Have fun!

food	grams of fat per serving	calories per serving	score fat (gm) X 9 ÷ calories
1. non-fat milk	_____	_____	_____
2. 2% fat milk	_____	_____	_____
3. whole milk	_____	_____	_____
4. mayonnaise	_____	_____	_____
5. diet mayonnaise	_____	_____	_____
6. crackers	_____	_____	_____
7. bread	_____	_____	_____
8. cheese	_____	_____	_____
9. reduced fat cheese	_____	_____	_____
10. _____	_____	_____	_____
11. _____	_____	_____	_____
12. _____	_____	_____	_____

Circle all of the foods above that are lighter foods (that have a score of 30 or lower)!

52

5. MATT'S MAGIC WORDS

Matt sat in Ms. Bacon's class the next morning with his shoulders hunched forward, his head hung low and his face filled with a frown. He looked like he had lost his best friend, like his fluffy white cat had been run over and like nobody had remembered his birthday. Matt looked glum.

He reached into his pocket when Ms. Bacon wasn't looking, searching until he found the chocolate covered peanut butter candy. He curled his fingers around the candy and waited. Ms. Bacon turned to the blackboard to explain a division problem. Matt's hand darted from his pocket to his mouth. His teeth crunched the brittle chocolate coating and his tongue relished the creamy peanut butter filling. He began to feel a shade, a tad, a bit less glum.

Cindy, Amy and Jesse watched as Matt's hand slid slowly into his pocket again. They watched his glum face relax as he popped another piece of chocolate covered peanut butter candy into his down-turned mouth. They could hear him crunch on the brittle chocolate coating and could imagine the creamy peanut butter swirling around his mouth.

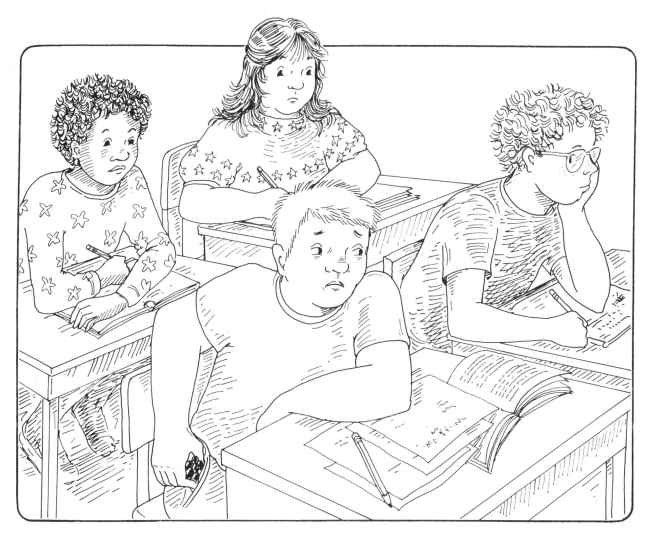

53

Just then Clown appeared on Matt's shoulder. Cindy jumped, "Clown, they'll see you. Ms. Bacon will, I know it!"

But Clown just smiled his easy smile and winked at her. And then in his most gentle voice replied, "But Cindy, my dear, your friend, Matt, is sad and is using food to try to cure his sadness."

"Clown," said Cindy, "The whole world cures sadness with food. Why should Matt be any different?"

"But my dear Cindy," replied Clown, "Food doesn't cure sadness, madness, boredom, anxiety or even loneliness. Food cures hunger. Why do you think he has to eat five handfuls of chocolate covered peanut butter candy? Because food is not very good at making bad feelings go away."

Cindy thought for a moment, "You mean, choose a solution that fits the problem?"

With that Clown jumped from Matt's shoulder, did a double somersault onto Matt's desk, "Whoopee, you got it, Cindy!"

Cindy scratched her head, twirled her hair around her index finger and continued, "So you cure sadness by crying, madness by punching a pillow, boredom by getting busy, anxiety by relaxing in a hot bath, and loneliness by calling a friend?"

Clown smiled affectionately at Cindy, "You can also cure difficult feelings by opening up and talking about them. When you talk about how you feel, it doesn't seem so bad. And you can discover ways to fix the feelings, too."

Clown was so thrilled and proud of his wis-dom that his nose started to glow. Matt, Amy and Cindy caught a glimpse of the glow. No one else besides the kids in the cozy corner of Ms. Baker's room could see Clown.

"Okay, Clown, I heard what you said. Are you making fun of me?" said Matt threateningly.

Clown quivered with fear. "Oh no, Matt. I'd never make fun of anybody bigger than a cookie jar!"

Matt's face softened, "I don't know how to open up, Clown. I do know how to spell Mississippi, read Dicken's stories and solve some algebra problems. But opening up — I just don't know the ABC's of it. When I feel bad, I usually just eat."

Clown looked at the four kids in the cozy corner, "Does anybody here know the magic words of how to open up?"

Cindy twirled her hair. Amy thought with the tip of her tongue at the corner of her mouth. There was a crease down the middle of Jesse's forehead that touched his glasses.

Ms. Bacon put up another set of math problems on the board. They thought some more . . . the magic words of how to open up . . . what could they be?

"I know," said Amy, jumping up. "The magic words are 'I feel . . .' and then you put after that whatever you feel!"

"So, instead of eating five handfuls of chocolate covered peanut butter candy, I could write a note to Cindy that said, "I feel sad."

"Exactly," agreed Clown, "and you could tell her what you were sad about."

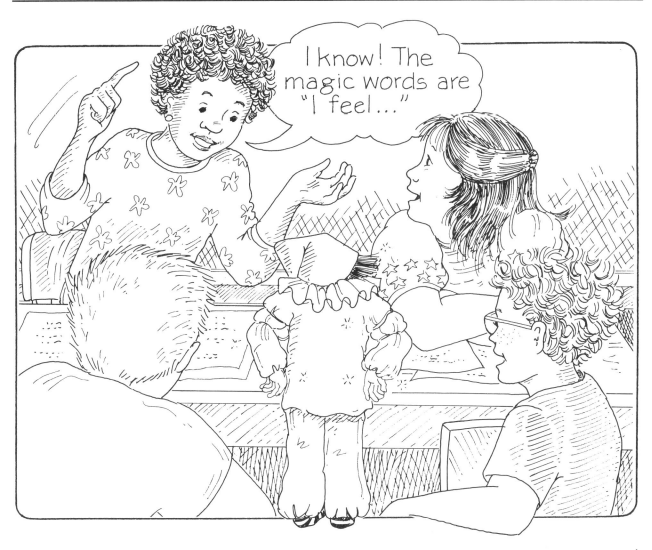

"That's difficult," replied Matt, "Lots of times I'm not sure what I'm sad about. In fact, I'm not absolutely sure it's sadness. I'm feeling a little mad, too."

"Terrific, Matt," beamed Clown, "You don't need to know what you're feeling or why before you open up. As you talk about it you learn more about your feelings and you try to figure out why you're feeling that way."

"You mean," said Amy, "You just start with the magic words, 'I feel .' and see what comes out?"

"That's exactly right, my sweet face," said Clown.

Matt looked up at the ceiling, down at the floor, "I feeeeeeeel . . . ." He looked through the windows to the birch trees past the fence, "I feel sad and angry and confused . . . "

"That's right, that's exactly right, Matt" said Clown. "Those are your feelings. You have a right to those feelings. Nobody can say you are wrong to feel that way. If you feel it, you feel it. That's it. Now . . . what are you feeling sad, angry and confused about?"

"I don't know," said Matt staunchly. "I just don't know."

"Try harder, Matt. What do you think you feel sad, angry and confused about?" said Amy. "Guess!"

"I feel sad, angry and confused because I'm

making changes. I'm eating lighter—except for today—exercising more and I've lost 3 pounds of fat. That's 12 cubes of butter, you know. But my mother and father are still stuck to the television and still pouring on the chips, salami and ice cream. It isn't fair."

"I know, Matt," said Cindy, "Talk to them. Tell them how you feel. Tell them what you want. They can always turn you down, but there's no chance that they'll do what you want unless you tell them what you want."

"What do you want, Matt?" asked Clown.

"I want to go on family hikes. I want my dad to play catch and soccer with me. I'd like to be not the only one using the trampoline while the television's on," said Matt.

Clown smiled his wide smile, "You did it, Matt. You opened up and talked about your feelings. You used the magic words, 'I feel . . .' and decided what you want. You are a star!"

"Yeah, you're a star, Matt!" shouted Cindy.

The room went quiet. Ms. Bacon's eyes turned red with anger, "Cindy, Matt, Amy and Jesse, I feel that your attention has drifted. It has drifted so far away that I'm not convinced that you understand these division problems. In fact, the only way I will be convinced is if you each do ten additional sets of math problems for your homework tonight."

So as Clown faded very slowly until only his broad smile remained, the kids in Ms. Bacon's cozy corner thought about the magic words, "I feel . . ." and the ten sets of math problems that were due the next day.

SMART TALK

Managing difficult feelings—You feel down. You're upset. You go to the cookie jar but know that you really aren't hungry. Eating those cookies won't make you feel up; they won't make you feel better.

Almost any difficult feeling can trigger some kids to eat. They have learned to eat when they feel sad, mad, bored, worried or lonely. When they feel especially bad inside they can eat a whole bag of cookies.

Eating to stuff away difficult feelings doesn't work. Think of difficult feelings as big, locked doors. On the other side of the doors are happy, peaceful feelings. To open the door you must find the right key.

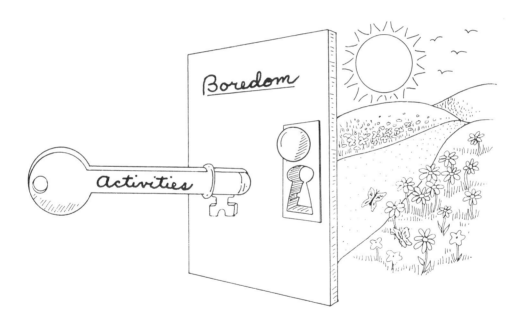

The only key that opens the door of loneliness and gets rid of all those difficult feelings is the key of people. Being with people you like opens the door of loneliness and brings you into the meadow of happy, peaceful feelings.

The only key that opens the door of boredom is the key of activities. Doing something you enjoy shoos away boredom and opens the door to happy, peaceful feelings.

Food only opens the door of hunger. When you use the key of food on your doors of sadness, anger, boredom, anxiety or loneliness, it doesn't work. While you're eating you don't think about your difficult feelings. But as soon as you stop eating, the difficult feelings come back. The door slams shut and you are closed off once again from happy, peaceful feelings.

SMART TALK continued

When you feel badly stop everything. You are important. The fact that you aren't feeling well matters. Think about how you are feeling. Figure out what you need to make yourself feel better. Find the "key" that fits your lock. Here are some examples of healthy ways to make difficult feelings better:

Open up and talk about your problem — Keeping it inside just makes things worse. Talk with your friend, parent, neighbor, teacher, dog, cat or anyone you trust. Talking about it helps you figure out what the problem is and gives you ideas for solving it.

Tell people how you feel — You have a right to how you feel. Nobody can tell you that your feelings are wrong. Talk about your feelings. Getting your feelings out is a big relief. Just start your sentences with the magic words "I feel . . . " and keep talking.

If people don't listen to you, tell them — Lots of times parents don't know how to listen very well. If you don't feel like they are listening to you, tell them. Politely say, "I don't feel listened to."

Write it out — What if there is no one to talk to? Get a notebook and make your own journal. Write down your fears, worries and secrets. It helps!

Move your body — Exercise lifts your spirits and makes the sad and mad monsters go away. Get some exercise to make your outlook happier.

Relax for a few minutes — Take some time just for yourself. Lie down on your bed. Breathe deeply and let your mind feel calm and relaxed.

Say good things to yourself — Be sure that the voice inside is friendly and encouraging. All day long you talk to yourself. Be sure that this "self-talk" is positive and loving. Say to yourself, "I'll be fine," "It will work out," or "It's okay not to be perfect." Be your own best friend.

Matt was feeling awful. How did he know that he felt awful? He noticed that after school he was starving. All he could think about was food. So he lay down on his bed and relaxed. He needed time to think. "I am feeling . . . . . worried." Good, that was a first step. But he didn't know what he was worried about. Matt called his mother at work. "Mom, I'm feeling worried but I don't know what I'm worried about." They talked for a while and Matt realized that he was worried about school. He hadn't been getting his homework done on time. Matt and his Mom figured out a way that he could get more time for homework.

Matt found that the door blocking good feelings was worry and that the key to unlock-

---

SMART TALK continued

ing that door was more time for homework. They only way he figured it out was by starting with the magic words, "I feel . . .

Cindy found herself thinking about sweets all the time. She usually thought about food when she had difficult feelings. Cindy walked out the front door and around the back garden where Grandpa was weeding around the tulips and the daffodils. "Grandpa," said Cindy, "I feel awful."

"So do I," Grandpa replied, "it's my back that bothers me, especially when I garden. Now pick up that hoe and get busy."

"Grandpa," said Cindy loudly, "I don't feel listened to. I have some bad feelings and I want to talk about them."

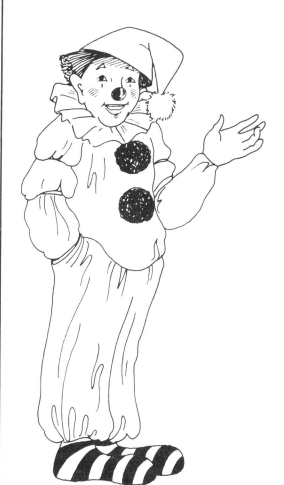

Grandpa looked up from his weeding, "Okay, Cindy, I'm listening."

Cindy started, "I feel . . . I don't know what I feel . . . I feel sad about Mom and Dad's divorce. It's been a while, but I still feel sad about it. And besides, Mom has no time to spend with me any more." Cindy continued talking until she realized that she should talk to her Mom about it directly.

That night at bedtime Cindy told her mother that she was still sad about the divorce and that she needed more time to spend with her. Her mom started crying and said that she missed time with Cindy, too. They agreed to take Sunday afternoons off to do something fun together.

Cindy found that the door blocking happy, peaceful feelings was sadness. The key opening that door was spending more time with her mother. Besides, she felt better just having talked to Grandpa and Mom about it rather than keeping it all bottled up inside.

─────SMART TALK continued─────

FOUR FOOD GROUPS

GROUP	SERVINGS	FOODS	SERVING SIZE
Milk	3	milk	8 ounces
		yogurt	8 ounces
		cottage cheese	1½ cups
		cheese	1 slice
Meat	2	beans, lentils	1 cup
		chicken or fish	1 piece
		meat	3 ounces
		nuts	¼ cup
		eggs	2
Vegetables and Fruit*	4	fruit	1 piece
		vegetables	¾ cup
Grain	4	bread	1 slice
		tortilla	1
		rice or pasta	½ cup
		pizza crust	1 piece

*try to include a citrus fruit or juice and a dark leafy green vegetable or yellow fruit/vegetable daily.

─────────────────

Eating well—Your body needs more than 50 nutrients to be healthy. You can get all of these building blocks of good health from eating a variety of foods from the Four Food Groups.

You can get a rough idea of how well you're doing at getting the nutrition your body needs by using the Four Food Groups system. The chart above lists the foods in each group, the size of a serving and the least amount of servings from each group you need.

A good rule of thumb is to have servings from all four groups at lunch and dinner and to have servings from at least three groups at breakfast.

YOUR TURN!

1. Matt and Cindy have decided to learn more about their feelings. They want to stop eating to stuff away difficult feelings. By figuring out their feelings they will be able to find the "key" that fits the lock and open the door to happy, peaceful feelings. Which of these feelings have you had in the last week? (check all that are true for you):

_____ sad   _____ angry

_____ mad   _____ worried

_____ lonely   _____ tired

_____ embarrassed   _____ hungry

_____ happy   _____ depressed

_____ bored   _____ anxious

_____ hurt   _____ confused

2. Name one of the feelings you have often:

_____

3. What do you do when you feel this way? (check all that are true for you):

_____ keep it to myself/don't say anything   _____ hit somebody or something

_____ talk to a friend   _____ hurt myself

_____ talk to my mother   _____ watch television

_____ talk to my father   _____ listen to music

_____ talk to my brother of sister   _____ do homework

_____ talk to another close friend/relative   _____ get busy doing something

_____ write down my feelings   _____ eat some food

_____ exercise   _____ cry

_____ relax by myself for a few minutes   _____ fight with my brother, sister or friend

_____ say good things to myself   _____ other_____

4. What do you plan to do next time you feel this way?

5. Most people feel difficult feelings every day. The next two times you feel badly, pause and figure out exactly how you are feeling. Write the feeling on the door below. Then figure out what you need to feel better. Write that on the key below. For instance, if Matt felt bored, he would write "bored" on the door below. If what he needed was an activity to interest him, he would write "activity" on the key. Now it's your turn!

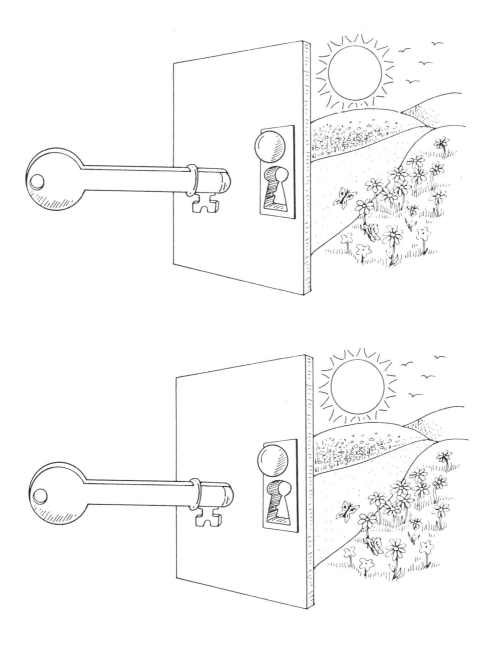

6. Name two people to whom you will start talking more often about how you feel:

_____

7. Look at the FOOD SUMMARY at the back of this book. List four FREE FOODS or LIGHT FOODS you like from each of the Four Food Groups.

Milk Group 1. _____

2. _____

3. _____

4. _____

Meat Group 1. _____

2. _____

3. _____

4. _____

Vegetable/ 1. _____
Fruit Group
2. _____

3. _____

4. _____

Grain Group 1. _____

2. _____

3. _____

4. _____

STICKER STROKES

Check if I did it!

Each day I will:

Take SHAPEDOWN TIME.

Write down my exercise.

Eat only FREE FOODS and LIGHT FOODS at lunch.

Take time to picture my body lean.

Exercise for 60 minutes or more.

Watch no TV until after I exercise, and limit TV to one hour.

My choice: _____

	MON.	TUES.	WED.	THURS.	FRI.	SAT.	SUN.

Number of goals I met:

My reward or privilege for making at least five goals every day this week is: _____ .

My weight: Start of the week _____   End of the week _____

My reward or privilege Goal

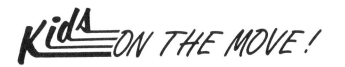

KIDS ON THE MOVE!

	MINUTES	ACTIVITY
MONDAY		
TUESDAY		
WEDNESDAY		
THURSDAY		
FRIDAY		
SATURDAY		
SUNDAY		

---JUST FOR FUN!---

MAKE CHEESE!

That's right. Be your own cheesemaker! Make your own batch of pot cheese. Pot cheese is a creamy smooth cheese made from yogurt that spreads on breads and makes great sandwiches. So put on your baker's hat and get started!

Gather your materials:

Unbleached muslin, a thin cotton dish towel or doubled cheese cloth—one half yard

String—one yard long

Plain yogurt (low-fat)—one quart or four 8- ounce containers

Make your cheese:

Place the yogurt in the middle of your cloth.

Bring the corners of the cloth up and tie a string around them to make a little "bag" of yogurt.

Hang the bag by tying it to your faucet over your sink.

Let the whey drip into your sink overnight.

The next morning spoon the pot cheese from the cloth into a bowl.

Enjoy your cheese:

Toast a piece of whole wheat bread.

Spread it with some pot cheese.

Eat it just like that or add a topping:
    a sprinkle of cinnamon   a dab of raspberry jam
    a layer of sliced strawberries   applesauce and nutmeg
    mild chile salsa or taco sauce   grated carrots
    thinly sliced apple

Rate your cheese: not good   good   great

6. SKATE BOARD MANIA

At recess Cindy and Amy were walking on the pathway to the office. Just as they came around the corner David crashed into them — and bowled them over. The girls fell to the pavement and David crashed to the ground. His skateboard kept careening down the path until it hit a prickly bush, rolled end over end, only stopping when it smashed into the plum tree that shaded the office.

Cindy's ankle burned! Little shavings of skin — like tissue paper — covered the wound on her ankle. Behind the white shavings bright red blood threatened to pour through the skin. "A bad scrape," thought Cindy. She looked over at Amy crying and rubbing her right knee.

Amy yelled at David, "Look what you did! Look what happened to my knee!" A drop of blood rolled down her shin from the deep gash below her knee cap.

David hung his head, found his skateboard and went on skating, this time a little more slowly. Amy turned to Cindy, "I feel so angry! He didn't even apologize! He didn't care that he hurt us! I can't believe how rude he was. And just think, he's going to get away with it! I feel so

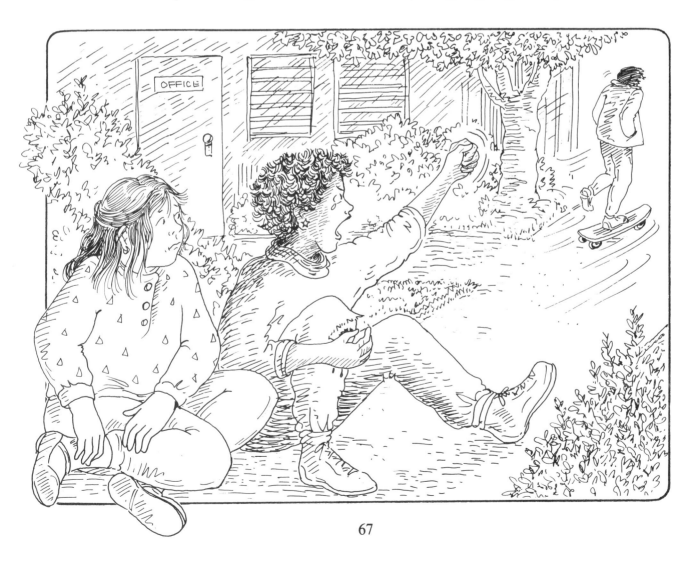

frustrated and powerless! He bloodies my body and gets off scot-free!"

Cindy nodded her head and said nothing.

Amy continued, "No, he's not going to get off scot-free. I'm going to tell Sophia at the office. She'll know what to do." Amy stomped off to the office.

Cindy stood next to the bushes. She didn't know how she felt. She didn't know what to say. The only thing she felt for sure was hungry. Maybe she didn't feel exactly starving but she definitely wanted something to eat. Food would help.

Wait. Cindy thought of the magic words, "I feel. . ." How she felt mattered. She sat down on the bench and thought, "How do I feel?"

Just then Clown popped onto her shoulder and did a front flip onto the pavement, "That's a good question, Cindy, how do you feel?"

"Not good."

"That's a start. How else do you feel?" said Clown.

"I feel bad about being quiet. I should have said what Amy said. I was mad. I did feel hurt. I wanted David to at least say he was sorry," said Cindy looking down at the pavement. A bluejay hopped along the pavement looking for bread crusts, found one and then flew away. Her eyes followed the bird as it flew up to the plum tree where he landed and quickly gulped down his bounty.

Clown thought. At times like this he wished he were only a silent cookie jar. He knew Cindy felt badly, but didn't know just what to say to her. Finally, Clown leaned forward, "Why didn't you say something, Cindy?"

"Because . . . " she said, watching the bluejay hop onto the lunch table, pick up a stray apple core and fly up over the office roof and out of sight.

"Because, why?" probed Clown, still feeling somewhat timid.

"Because, if I did say what was on my mind, David would have teased me. He has the biggest mouth at school. He loves to laugh at me and call me fat-so or tub-o."

Cindy burst into tears — big tears, the kind that jump out of your eyes and run to the ground and make big wet drops on the pavement. She held her head in her hands and wept some more.

Now Clown really wished he were just a cookie jar. He didn't care what kind of cookie jar. A soldier would be fine. Even a pig cookie jar would do, just so that he wouldn't have to see Cindy looking so sad.

Cindy looked up at Clown's mournful face, "Clown, what are you feeling?"

"I'm feeling sad . . . and helpless. I want to help you feel better but I don't know how," answered Clown.

Cindy smiled and brushed away the last tear.

Clown shook his head and a smile suddenly appeared on his face just like a light bulb turning on, "I know! Listen to me right now, Cindy. We have some serious talking to do."

"We do?" asked Cindy.

"We certainly do," replied Clown. "David was rude, but you were passive. You hung back and

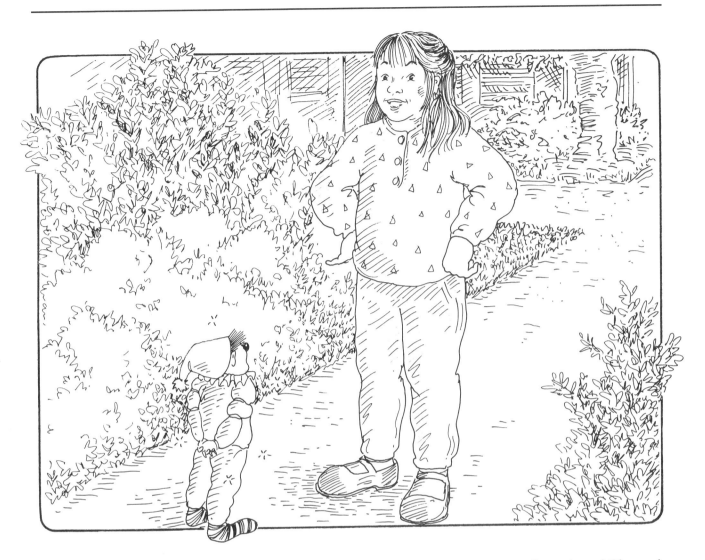

didn't say what you thought. You didn't tell anybody how they could help you, either. You need to spit it out and tell people your thoughts, feelings and needs—to speak up rather than to clam up."

"I know, and I'm doing better at it than I used to. But David is right when he says I'm fat and ugly. It hurts me so much when he says it," replied Cindy, with another tear threatening to fall from her eye.

"Oh," said Clown, "I get it. All that matters is whether you're fat or skinny. If the scale goes up you're ugly, and if it goes down you're not. How you look is based on weight and that's it."

"Maybe." replied Cindy.

"And your appearance," continued Clown, is all that matters. You are how you look. Nobody cares whether you're kind, funny, loving, honest, courageous, hard-working, or talented."

Cindy got up.

Clown went on, "So let's just line up all the kids in your class one after another. We'll weigh each one and then we'll line them up in order of their weight. The ones that weigh the least will get awards for being great people and the ones that weigh the most will be given awful people awards."

Cindy laughed, "You're right. It's dumb. Even if he calls me fat-so it hurts but it doesn't hurt that much. He's just acting rude. He's really a pest. Everybody knows it. If he keeps acting pesty he'll have no friends left at all."

Clown was relieved. He let out a huge sigh.

"And you're right on another thing, Clown," said Cindy, "I like my body. Sure, I'm losing some of my extra fat, but even if I were fat forever it doesn't mean I'm ugly. It just means I have more fat than other people do. I still have pretty blue eyes, a nice smile, pink cheeks, strong legs, and smooth skin."

Clown nodded. "You're right, Cindy, even if I stay a little bit scrawny my whole life my body will still be very lovable. See this nose? How could I ever wish or hope for a better nose than this? Even Cousin Owl's nose is not straighter or more perfectly shaped," he said lifting his nose in the air and touching it gingerly.

"Clown, you sound like all that matters is how you look. Is that all you are, a ceramic pot of a cookie jar?" demanded Cindy.

"Why no, Cindy, I have lots of good qualities," said Clown hesitantly.

"Sure you do. You know when to talk and when to be quiet. You care about people — and other cookie jars — and you do great flips!" observed Cindy with a slow smile forming on her lips.

"Thanks, Cindy," said Clown and his white skin turned to a rose colored blush. Clown stood up very straight, coughed three times and said, "Okay, Cindy, it's your turn. It's easy to see the good qualities in other people. It's harder to see them in yourself. Name three of your good qualities."

"Oh, that's easy," replied Cindy confidently. She paused. She scratched her head. She looked around for that bluejay. He must have headed off to another playground.

"I'm listening . . " prompted Clown.

"Let's see, " said Cindy, "I'm funny."

"That's one."

"I'm . . . honest," Cindy continued.

"Just one more."

"I'm good at talking about my feelings!" Cindy said proudly.

"Yes, you are, my not-so-round-fluffy-or-soft friend," laughed Clown. The bell rang. "Now what are you going to do?"

"I'm going to wash off this scrape and go to class," replied Cindy.

"What about David?" asked Clown as he began to slowly disappear.

"If I'm feeling mad I'll tell him so. I'm going to say what I think and tell him I want an apology. If he teases me about weight, I'll ignore him. I'd rather be round than rude and pesty. Besides, everybody gets teased about something. I wonder what kids will tease me about after I get the rest of this extra fat off? Oh, well, Clown . . . Clown, where did you go?"

Cindy could think of another thing good about Clown. He was smart. He was helping her love herself and her body and to speak up about her thoughts, feelings and needs. She'd have to remember to give him a hug for that!

SMART TALK

Speaking up — You've already learned how to speak up and say, "no thanks" to food. You've also started opening up and talking about your feelings. Now let's practice speaking up in other ways, like saying what you think and need, telling people how to help you, and talking about your problems.

When you talk about your thoughts, needs and problems you get something back. What is that something? You get more attention and affection. All that attention and affection make you feel more loved, safe and important. Those good feelings make you eat less. You stop using the key of food to unlock the door of feeling lonely, unloved and unimportant.

By speaking up, you help the people who love you learn more about how to give you the attention and affection you need. This is a habit you can use your whole life. When you grow up your friends, husband or wife and boss won't know what you need and what your problems are unless you tell them. So you can start this habit now and keep it for good.

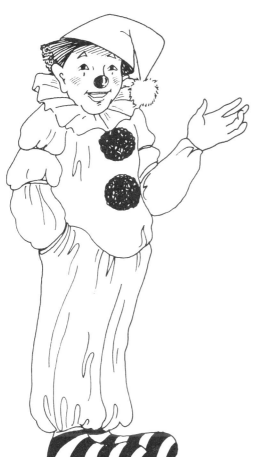

How do you do it? Just start your sentences with the magic phrases:

I feel . . . . .
I think . . . .
I need . . . . .
I have a problem about . . . .

Is speaking up rude? No. You are just stating your thoughts, feelings, needs and problems. That's not rude. You start your sentences with the word "I." This is important. Use "I" sentences. Watch the difference. Which sentence is rude?

I need a new tennis racquet.

You have to get me a tennis racquet.

That's right, the "I" sentence is not rude. The "you" sentence is. Your thoughts, feelings, needs are important. You have a right to have them and by using "I" sentences you can tell others your thoughts, feelings and needs without being rude.

71

SMART TALK continued

Handling put-downs — Nobody likes people teasing them. It hurts. You probably don't like it when people tease you about weight. You feel ashamed and embarrassed. You feel differently. What can you do about put-downs? Think about the idea that it happens to almost everybody. Everybody is different in some way — taller, shorter, fatter, thinner. In fact, once you get the extra fat off your body there will probably be some person at school who will tease you about something else.

Think about the poor person who is saying those things. He or she is rude and pesty and doesn't have many friends. That person also probably feels ashamed of being so hurtful and rude. Aren't you glad that you are not hurtful, rude and pesty?

Most of the time, it's best to ignore the put-downs when they happen. Pretend that you didn't hear what they said. They probably won't keep on teasing you unless they know that it bothers you. Just turn and walk away. Later talk to your mom, dad and other person close to you and tell them how you feel. If you feel hurt, sad or embarrassed, tell them how you feel.

If your brother, sister or best friend teases you or if someone at school is teasing you very badly, speak up and talk to your mom or dad. Tell them about your problem. You should not have to put up with lots of put-downs. They will help you solve it.

With certain people it pays to speak up to put-downs. Let's say, for instance, that your brother or sister is teasing you. That hurts you every day. Speak up and say, "I feel hurt when you say that."

Liking your body — Some people think that the only thing that's important is how they look. If they don't look "perfect" they hate themselves. If they aren't at a "perfect" weight, they think they are a failure. They are afraid to get on the scale because they will feel like a bad person if they weight too much. What a sad way to live, never accepting and loving your body — imperfections and all.

A happier, healthier attitude is that your weight is only one part of how you look. And how you look is only one part of you. Bodies come in many sizes and shapes. Whatever its size and shape, your body is likable and lovable. You probably have some favorite parts of your body. Everybody does. And you probably have some parts you don't like as well. Everybody else does, too.

Take five minutes of ME TIME each day to think about the things that you like about your wonderful body. That way you can develop good feelings about your body Keep in mind the things you like about yourself that have nothing to do with how you look. Think about how kind you are, how smart you are, how truthful you are, how well you shoot baskets or remember your lines for a play. Be "up" about yourself!

YOUR TURN!

1. Cindy is going to speak up more often. She will talk to her mom and grandpa about her problems. Check off all the problems you have now. If some of my problems aren't listed, add them to the bottom of the list.

_____ getting out of bed on time

_____ getting to school on time

_____ remembering to bring home my jacket

_____ remembering to bring home my homework

_____ doing my homework on time

_____ not doing well in school

_____ not having anyone to play with

_____ having an argument with a friend

_____ other kids teasing me

_____ remembering to exercise after school

_____ not eating too much with friends

_____ arguing with my brother or sister

_____ feeling sad about mom and dad arguing

_____ feeling worried about money

_____ eating too much after school

_____ feeling worried about someone who is sick

_____ feeling upset about someone who died

_____ feeling lonely

_____ feeling bored

_____ feeling angry

_____ feeling sad

_____ feeling like I don't get enough attention from mom

_____ feeling like I don't get enough attention from dad

_____ feeling sad about not seeing one of my parents enough

_____ feeling afraid of someone hurting me

_____ feeling ashamed or worried about a secret

_____ other problems:_____

_____

When you speak up, you talk to someone about your troubles. You tell them what you think, feel, and need. Pick two of the problems you checked above and talk to someone about them.

Remember to use the magic words: I feel, I think, I need, I have a problem.

One of my problems: _____

    To whom I will talk: _____

    What I will tell them: _____

_____

_____

    Did I speak up?   yes   no   unsure

Another of my problems: _____

    To whom I will talk: _____

    What I will tell them: _____

_____

_____

    Did I speak up?   yes   no   unsure

2. Who teases you about your weight?

_____

Check what you will do about these put-downs:

_____ Think that everybody gets teased about something.

_____ Think that the person is rude and a pest, has few friends and is probably ashamed for being so hurtful.

_____ Keep quiet at the time and afterward talk to my mom or dad about my hurt feelings.

_____ Keep quiet at the time and afterward talk to my mom or dad and ask them to help me get them to stop teasing me.

_____ Speak up to the person and tell him or her that what they say hurts my feelings.

_____ Something else: _____

3. Name five things about how you look that you like:

    1. _____

    2. _____

    3. _____

    4. _____

    5. _____

4. Name three things you have done that you are proud of:

    1. _____

    2. _____

    3. _____

5. Name three of your good qualities — things you like about yourself like your sense of humor, your kindness to people, your honesty, your generosity, your voice, your strength, your gracefulness, and so on.

    1. _____

    2. _____

    3. _____

Each day I will:

Take SHAPEDOWN TIME.

Write down my breakfast.

Eat only fruits and veggies for snacks.

Take ME TIME to think about good things about myself.

Exercise for 60 minutes or more.

Watch no TV until after I exercise, and limit TV to one hour.

My choice: _____

Number of goals I met:

My reward or privilege for making at least five goals every day this week is: _____ .

My weight: Start of the week _____ Goal _____ End of the week _____

STICKER STROKES

Check if I did it!

	MON.	TUES.	WED.	THURS.	FRI.	SAT.	SUN.

MY BREAKFAST

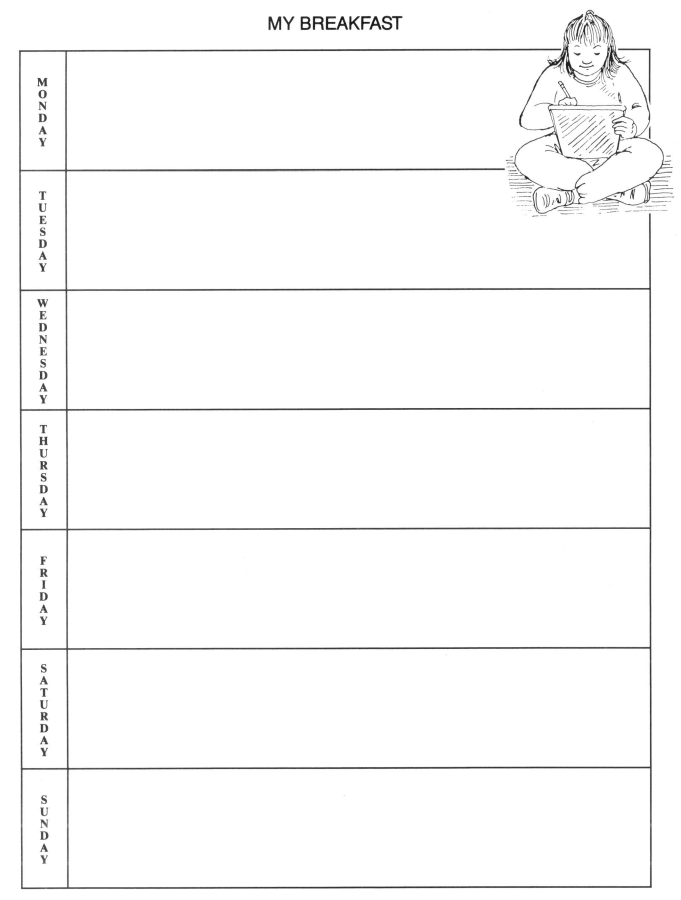

MONDAY	
TUESDAY	
WEDNESDAY	
THURSDAY	
FRIDAY	
SATURDAY	
SUNDAY	

Number of days I ate mainly LIGHT FOODS and FREE FOODS_____

Number of days I ate foods from at least three of the Four Food Groups_____

JUST FOR FUN!

FUN WITH FRUITS

Circle the kinds of fruit in the puzzle below. Can your find all 12 of them? (4 are on the diagonal)

```
A   G   U   A   V   A   D   C

C   P   A   P   A   Y   A   I

A   O   P   E   A   R   T   V

S   M   R   L   I   M   E   M

A   D   E   A   E   P   S   A

B   S   G   L   N   N   O   N

A   I   C   H   O   G   E   G

F   S   P   R   U   N   E   O
```

Name one kind of fruit you will try this week. Try it and then describe it.

Fruit I will eat this week:_____

How this fruit looked, smelled and tasted:_____

My three favorite kinds of fruit: 1. _____

2. _____

3. _____

7. MATT'S CRAVINGS

Matt sat in the cozy corner reading about the Boston Tea Party. He wanted a tea party, too. Or make it a pizza party. Or an ice cream bash. Yes, that would do. An ice cream bash with six flavors of ice cream, hot fudge, marshmallow sauce and butterscotch topping, maybe some nuts and cherries and definitely gobs of whipped cream. After two months of turkey on whole wheat bread, apples and bananas he was ready for a diet revolt.

Matt wrote a note to Cindy and slipped across to her when Ms. Baker left the room to take Nathan, who had just thrown up, to Sophia at the office to call his parents. Cindy opened the note slowly. It said, "Dear SHAPEDOWN buddy, I know I'm getting in shape and I really like it but I feel like a food revolt right now. I want to go on the rampage and eat everything in sight. Your friend, Matt."

Cindy sighed. Uh oh. Here Matt goes again, thought Cindy. Another pizza and ice cream binge was in the making. For the last two months Matt had looked so happy. He had brought LIGHT FOODS to school for lunch. He had played football a lot and had been running faster. He even had been making some touchdowns.

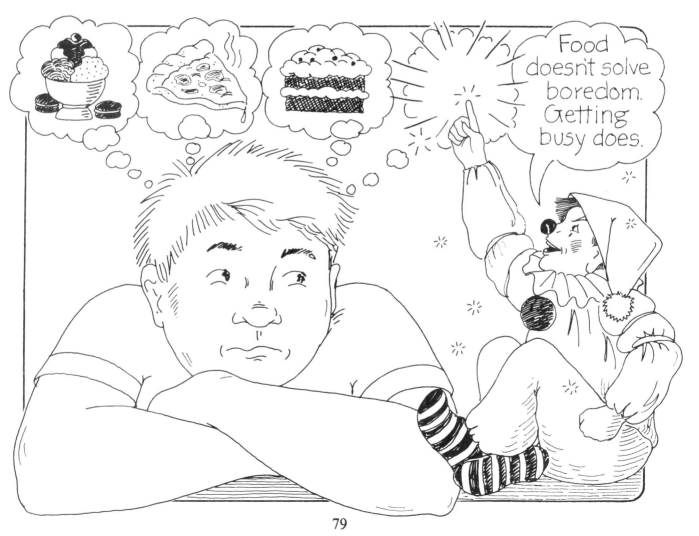

The other boys always wanted to play with him now. Matt had to do something to keep himself from blowing it.

Cindy wrote back, "You're just having a craving. It will pass. Think about how great it feels to make those touchdowns," and she passed her note to Matt just as Ms. Bacon entered the room.

Matt slid the note into the middle of his opened history book. When Ms. Bacon went back to grading papers he carefully snuck the note from his book and unfolded and read it. Cindy didn't understand, thought Matt. He **really** craved ice cream. It had been building in him for a whole month. Yesterday he had even snuck a candy bar from his father's top drawer. Now he wanted more.

"Snuck a candy bar, huh?" said a voice. Clown appeared, perched on Matt's pencil rack.

"Yes," replied Matt, looking down at the pencil he was twirling.

"What made you decide to have a candy bar?" asked Clown.

"I felt deprived. I haven't had candy in two months," said Matt "and I was feeling bored and lonely after school."

"Food doesn't solve boredom, getting busy does. It doesn't solve sadness, or anger either. The thing that it solves well is hunger. Just like water solves thirst. Did sneaking the candy bar make you feel better?" asked Clown.

"Yes. I mean no. I liked the sweet chocolate taste, but that only lasted about 90 seconds. Then I felt worse. I was mad at myself. And disappointed. Sneaking feels like lying. It feels bad," replied Matt.

"If you decide to eat a candy bar, just eat it.

Don't feel guilty. Don't sneak," said Clown.

"But if my parents knew I ate a candy bar they'd be red hot mad," replied Matt.

"Untrue. False. Wrong. Your parents love you. They care more about you than about how fat you are. If you're feeling deprived they will help you work out a way to eat a candy bar. But they can't help you unless you tell them how you are feeling," said Clown crossing his legs.

"You really mean it?" said Matt. Clown nodded. "That makes me relax inside. I can really talk with them about what I'm thinking and feeling! It's funny. I've stopped craving ice cream now that I know I can always work out a way to have it."

The bell rang. Clown disappeared instantly. Cindy approached Matt, "Let's talk, Matt."

"That's okay, Cindy. My cravings vanished. When I want something I can work out a way to get it."

"How?" asked Cindy.

"Trade-offs," replied Matt.

"Trade-offs?" questioned Cindy.

"Yes, like every once in a while when I crave an ice cream cone, I can eat only half a sandwich for lunch, then have my cone. That's a trade-off. I work them out with my parents during SHAPE-DOWN TIME. Easy, huh?"

"Yeah, easy," replied Cindy wondering what miracle had struck Matt.

"Can you come over after school tomorrow? We can go on a bike ride or play some tennis and then have dinner," said Cindy.

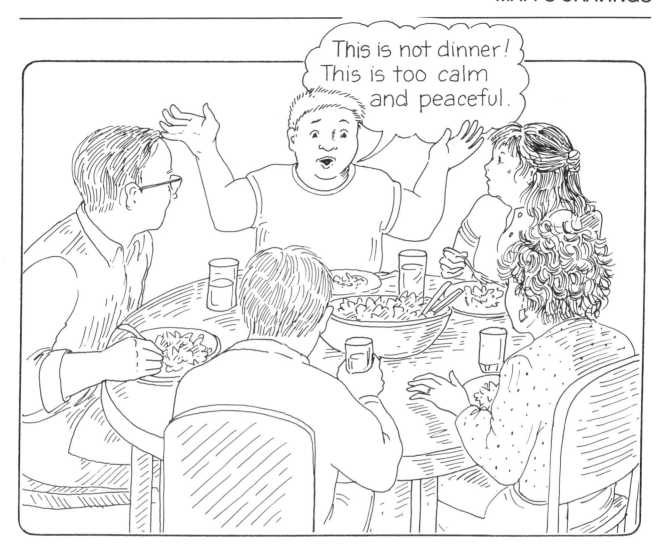

"Sounds great!" said Matt.

The next day after school Cindy and Matt rode on their bikes to Cindy's house. They hit tennis balls against the garage door, listened to music and then helped out with dinner. They set the table and made a salad, washing the lettuce, slicing the ripe, red tomatoes and the crisp cucumbers.

Finally, dinner was ready. They had a huge green salad with a little dressing sprinkled on top, a big baked potato with a tiny dab of butter and sliced turkey breast with cranberry sauce. Yummmmm.

Cindy's mom and grandpa, her half-brother Michael and Matt savored the hot turkey and crunched on the crisp salad. Cindy and her family talked about their days. What went well and what didn't and how they were feeling. It was peaceful and fun. Michael had followed a football into the bushes, right into a yellow jacket's nest and had been stung on the nose. Cindy's grandfather had won $5 in the lottery. Cindy had done better at math and had made a new friend at school named Nicola. Cindy's mom talked about the new secretary at work. She was from New York City and knew all about the new Broadway plays there. Matt was quiet.

Finally, he blurted out, "This is not dinner. This is too calm and peaceful. There's no television blaring, no people ignoring each other, no gulping down food. This is strange!"

There was a hush. Then mom spoke, "This is

how we like to eat. We're in the habit of enjoying our food and each other. On days when someone is grouchy or too tired, they talk about it. We try our best to make meals relaxing, a time we can be together."

"Oh," said Matt, "In my house we go and come as we please. The television's usually on. Sometimes we eat dinner. Other times we just snack all night."

"There's nothing wrong with that, Matt," said Michael. "If it works well for your family and doesn't make you eat too much, it's just fine."

"But when we snack instead of have dinner, I eat three bowls of cereal and half a box of crackers. And when I watch television and eat I don't even taste my food. I don't think it works that well."

So as Mom, Grandpa, Michael, Cindy and Matt had seconds on salad, Matt schemed about convincing his family to change their eating style. They cleared the dishes and Matt said his good-bye's and thank you's and walked home with the full moon pouring out white light that touched his face and made him feel peaceful. It had been a very good day.

SMART TALK

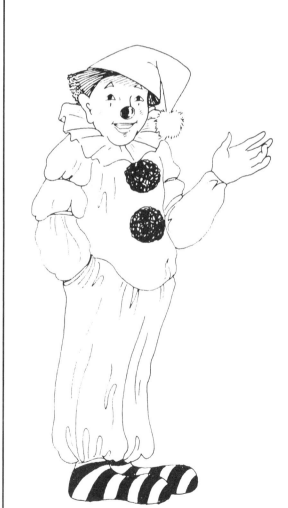

Cravings — Have you had cravings yet? Cravings are when your mouth wants something so badly that your brain can think of nothing else. If you have a chocolate craving you walk around with a chocolate bar glued to your brain. You keep thinking about that chocolate bar. You want chocolate and you want it right now! That's a craving.

What do you do about cravings? You find out what's causing them. What causes cravings? Several things. Habit is one cause. You're used to eating the food and now you miss it. Deprivation is another cause. You've been over-doing your healthy eating so you feel deprived. Another cause is hunger. If you're skipping meals or not eating enough at meals you may get so hungry that you crave foods. Still another is feelings. If you're feeling depressed, lonely or angry, you may crave sweets or breads. So the main reasons for cravings are habit, deprivation, hunger and feelings.

The solution to cravings is to tell your parent during SHAPEDOWN TIME that you are having a craving. Your parent will help you figure our what is causing your craving and help you find a solution. Here's what you can do about it, too:

Eat regular meals. Skipping meals just creates cravings. If you skip breakfast you'll feel starved by noon and crave JUNK FOODS.

Don't deprive yourself. No foods are always forbidden in SHAPEDOWN. Be sure to have your favorite food at least once a week.

Eat enough food. If your meals and snacks are too skimpy you'll get extra hungry and that hunger will fuel your cravings.

Eating secretly — Kids who eat secretly usually feel badly about it. They take a cookie from the cupboard and "steal" some chips from the drawer. Eating secretly feels like you are lying. You feel like you've done something very wrong. It's not all your fault, though. Your parents' job is to make you feel comfortable talking with them about difficult things like wanting food that you're not supposed to have. It really doesn't matter whose fault it is. What matters is that from now on whenever you feel like eating secretly, you talk to your parents about it.

Your parents will help you with cravings and secretive eating in many different ways. One way they will help you is by making up trade-offs. Every once in a while when you really want something — like an ice cream cone — they can help you figure out a way to eat less, eat lighter or exercise more the rest of the day so you can have it. Here are some examples of trade-offs:

Situation: Matt wanted to go to a birthday party and eat the cake, ice cream, hot dog and chips.

Trade-off: No dessert with dinner all week and two hours of exercise on the day of the party.

Situation: Cindy wanted to have a candy bar for an after school snack.

Trade-off: Half a sandwich and two baggies of veggies for lunch.

Eating style — What your family eats is your family nutrition. How they eat is your family eating style. There is an eating style that helps people enjoy their food more and feel more satisfied by their mealtimes. This eating style also helps them eat more healthfully.

A healthy family eating style is when parents and kids eat together at the same time and at the same table. Mealtime is about the same time every night. The television is off and nobody reads the newspaper. Everybody eats their food slowly and enjoys every bite. They talk about their feelings and say what's on their minds. They say what happened — both the good and the bad — in their lives that day. They don't talk about weight, eating, exercise or nutrition. They just enjoy the food they are eating. Parents don't urge the kids to eat or not to eat. Kids don't ask their parents how much they have to eat. This way of eating is good for both kids and parents and for both health and weight.

Eating cues — Cravings can be triggered by cues like hunger, feeling deprived or sadness. We call anything that triggers you to say to yourself, "I want something to eat" an eating cue.

Hunger can be a cue but often cues have nothing to do with hunger. Often people, places, favorite foods, situations and moods trigger eating. If these non-hunger cues trigger your eating often, you're likely to gain weight. So keeping you weight down means learning how not to let non-hunger cues trigger you to eat. Here are some cues that trigger kids to eat:

Food — The smell of fresh, warm chocolate chip cookies as you walk through the mall, the sight of a juicy cheeseburger on a television commercial and the cookie jar, chocked full of sugar cookies calling to your across the kitchen are all cues to eat. Seeing, tasting, thinking about and feeling food can make you want to eat it, particularly when its food that you like.

People — It's difficult when Grandma bakes up your favorite brownies, when Dad brings home doughnuts or when your best friend hands you a chocolate candy bar. These people can trigger you to eat food you don't need.

Places — Places can trigger you to eat even though you really aren't hungry. The sight of the school snack bar or of the doughnut shop may signal you to eat. Simply being in the kitchen can trigger your thoughts to turn to food.

Situations — Certain situations like holiday feasts and birthday parties. Perhaps being home alone triggers you to eat or going to the mall with friends is difficult. Baby-sitting or having snacks after the baseball game may trigger you to eat more than you need. When you're sick you may eat non-stop, starting with hot chocolate and then working your way through the graham cracker box.

Moods — Almost any mood can be a cue to eat. Feeling angry, bored, tired, sad, anxious, happy, excited, frustrated, lonely, unloved, disgusted or guilty can prompt you to eat when you aren't really hungry.

Times — Certain times of the day can trigger you to eat. You may eat dinner just because it's dinner time or have a snack after school just because it's 3:30 p.m. You may eat just because it's time to eat.

Everybody gets these eating cues. If you eat when you get these cues, you'll probably always be heavy. But just the way that you have learned to eat when you get these cues, you can learn not to eat when you get them. Here are several strategies for stopping cues before they trigger you to eat.

Blocking — Stop the cue dead in it's tracks. Keep it from reaching you. Keep out of the kitchen and away from food. Tell people not to offer you food. Put space between yourself and food.

SMART TALK continued

Pausing — Instead of eating when you get the urge to eat, stop and figure out your choices. Decide to do one of them.

STEP 1. Pause

STEP 2. Think of all your choices (including eating)

STEP 3. List the good and bad about each choice

STEP 4. Decide on one choice and do it

At lunchtime at school Amy offered Cindy a cookie. She paused and thought of her choices: To say "No thanks!", to take it and eat it or to take it and save it for her grandpa. If she said "No thanks!" it would help her lose weight but she wouldn't get to eat the cookie. If she took the cookie and ate it she would enjoy the cookie right then, but later she would wish she hadn't. If she saved it for grandpa, he would eat it and it wouldn't be good for him either. Cindy thought of her choices and the good and bad of each and decided to say "No thanks!"

Delaying — You can put off eating. Just put off eating the food for ten minutes. Say to yourself, "If I still want the food in ten minutes, I'll eat it then." Lots of times at the end of ten minutes you don't want the food anymore.

As you figure out what your cues are and manage them you learn a lot about your feelings and how to control your eating. A lot of these skills can be used in other things that you do, too.

YOUR TURN!

1. Matt's cravings for candy were triggered by feeling deprived. Cindy's cues are watching TV, feeling sad and her grandpa's brownies. Both Cindy and Matt are working on their family's eating style. Name a food you've had a craving for:

_____

2. Why do you think you get cravings? (Check all that are true for you.)

_____ habit — I'm used to having that food

_____ deprivation — having a too-healthy diet

_____ hunger — not eating enough

_____ feelings — like sadness, anger or boredom

3. What will you do the next time you have a craving?

_____

4. Name a food you've eaten secretly:

_____

5. What will you do the next time you want to eat secretly?

_____

6. Rate your family's eating style. Which of these things does your family already do at dinner time?

Your parent is in charge of:

what time your meals and snacks are	yes	sometimes	no
what foods are in your meals and snacks	yes	sometimes	no

You are in charge of:

whether or not you eat	yes	sometimes	no
how much of the food you eat	yes	sometimes	no

You turn off the television when you are eating	yes	sometimes	no
You get rid of books and newspapers when you are eating	yes	sometimes	no
You eat your food slowly, enjoying every bite	yes	sometimes	no
You talk freely about your feelings and thoughts	yes	sometimes	no
When you talk, people listen to you	yes	sometimes	no
You don't talk about weight, eating, exercise or nutrition	yes	sometimes	no
Parents as well as children enjoy the meal and the food	yes	sometimes	no
Parents do not urge their kids to eat or not to eat	yes	sometimes	no
Kids don't question their parents about what they have to eat	yes	sometimes	no

7. Describe the cues that trigger you to eat when you are really not hungry.

Moods_____

Times_____

People_____

Foods_____

Situations_____

Places_____

8. Pick one cue to manage by blocking, pausing or delaying, like blocking boredom after school by having friends over or blocking food cues by staying out of the kitchen.

Cue:_____

How I will manage it:_____

STICKER STROKES

Check if I did it!

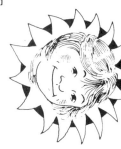

Each day I will:

Take SHAPEDOWN TIME.

Write down what I eat between 2 p.m. and dinner.

Eat breakfast, lunch and dinner.

Use a healthy family eating style at dinner.

Exercise for 60 minutes or more.

Watch no TV until after I exercise, and limit TV to one hour.

My choice: _____

	MON.	TUES.	WED.	THURS.	FRI.	SAT.	SUN.

Number of goals I met: _____ _____ _____ _____ _____ _____ _____

My reward or privilege for making at least five goals every day this week is: _____ .

My weight: Start of the week _____   Goal _____   End of the week _____

MY AFTERNOON SNACKS

MONDAY	
TUESDAY	
WEDNESDAY	
THURSDAY	
FRIDAY	
SATURDAY	
SUNDAY	

Number of days I had mainly FREE FOODS and LIGHT FOODS_____

MAGIC GARDEN SOUP

Cook vegetables to make a magic soup. Where is the magic? In the vegetables. Watch how they change when you cook them!

Gather your materials

2 onions
6 celery stalks
4 carrots
3 tomatoes
3 other kinds of vegetables of your choice!
4 bouillon cubes
paring knife
large sauce pan or kettle

Make your soup

Wash the vegetables well, cut them in one inch slices and place them in a very large, deep pan. Add two quarts of warm water and 4 bouillon cubes plus any herbs you like, such as parsley, bay or basil. Cook over low heat until the vegetables are tender. Watch the vegetables change their texture and shape. Where did the tomatoes go to? For fun, about 10 minutes before it's done, add ½ cup alphabet noodles.

Enjoy your Magic Garden Soup

Ladle up your soup. You made the magic!

What three kinds of vegetables did you use?

_____

_____

_____

8. CINDY'S AFTER SCHOOL ADVENTURE

Cindy sat in the cozy corner at the back of Ms. Bacon's class doing her math problems. She yawned. Math was boring and science dragged. She knew how to do everything there was to do on the playground. At home there was nothing worth doing but TV. She yawned again and quickly snapped her mouth closed as a fly buzzed past her nose. The fragrant spring air lazily drifted through the window rocking her to sleep.

Life was a little slow these days except for TV. In fact, life was boring. She thanked Mother Nature for the tube. Each afternoon she watched one favorite program after another. She wished that she could attach herself to the TV for good. Maybe a doctor could perform a complicated operation and then she'd never have to leave her beloved TV. Ever.

Matt was stuck on the third from the last math problem. He erased again. The paper shed little curls of paper. If he erased one more time he'd go clear through to the desk. Just then he caught a glimpse of Cindy, looking bored and restless. Cindy was looking leaner alright, but those bowls of candy cereal and the stacks of chocolate cookies she ate while watching the blaring tube didn't help.

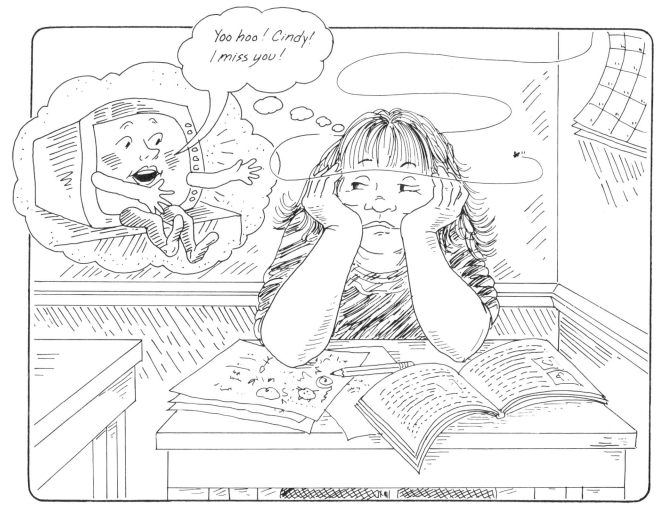

91

Cindy passed Matt a note, "Rescue me from this endless sea of boredom."

Matt chuckled and returned to the third to the last math problem.

Cindy passed another note, "Help, carry me to my television before I am snuffed out by the boredom monster."

Matt wrote, "Spend the afternoon with me and you'll ban boredom forever, that is, if you are brave enough!"

Matt slipped the note between the pages of his assignment book and tossed it onto Cindy's desk just as Ms. Bacon dropped her glasses on the floor and all the kids in the front row jumped up to retrieve them.

With a crooked smile on her expectant face, Cindy opened the assignment book and read Matt's challenge. Could she keep up with him all afternoon? Why not? Otherwise it would be the same old thing: television and candy cereal.

When the last bell rang, Cindy ran to find her backpack and raced up to Matt, "I'm ready," she said brightly, "but I'll bet you I'll be bored silly. My mind will wander to chocolate cookies and my candy cereal—the one with the little fruit flavored marshmallows in it."

Matt looked amused. "Just try not to be a slow poke!" he replied and hopped onto his bike. Cindy straddled her own and followed as Matt raced around the ivy-covered church and through the tunnel to the green lawn that stretched across the park. Matt jumped from his bike, grabbed a soccer ball and kicked it once, twice and then into the goal.

"One point for me," beamed Matt. "I'm going to beat you!"

"Wait! Stop!" said Cindy, putting the kick-stand down on her bike. The ball darted from her foot and the game was on.

When the score was four to four, Matt abruptly grabbed the ball and raced to his bike. "Beat you to my house!" he called.

His bike soared back through the tunnel, past the ivy-covered church, through the school yard and down the curvy street to his home with Cindy trailing all the way.

"Had enough?" Matt smiled.

"Never!" responded Cindy, her hair blowing in the wind and her cheeks flaming pink.

"Well, hold on!" he replied. Ralph, Matt's gray sheep dog sniffed at his heels. "It's bath time, my friend," said Matt and then grasped Ralph's collar, filled a tub with warm sudsy water and washed the dog until the water turned black and Ralph's white coat sparkled brightly.

Ralph emerged from the tub, looked straight into Cindy's eyes and shook. In one minute flat Cindy was soaked from head to food. She giggled. She laughed. She dropped to her knees, rolled on the grass and laughed some more. Ralph just licked her face.

Matt brought the wet towels into the house and found his mother's note. It read:

Matt,

Dinner tonight is fruit salad with vanilla yogurt and turkey sandwiches on whole wheat rolls. Will you pick up the freshest fruit and some non-fat yogurt at the store on your way home from karate class?

Thanks, Mom

P.S. Are we having foods from all Four Food Groups for dinner?

P.P.S. I love you.

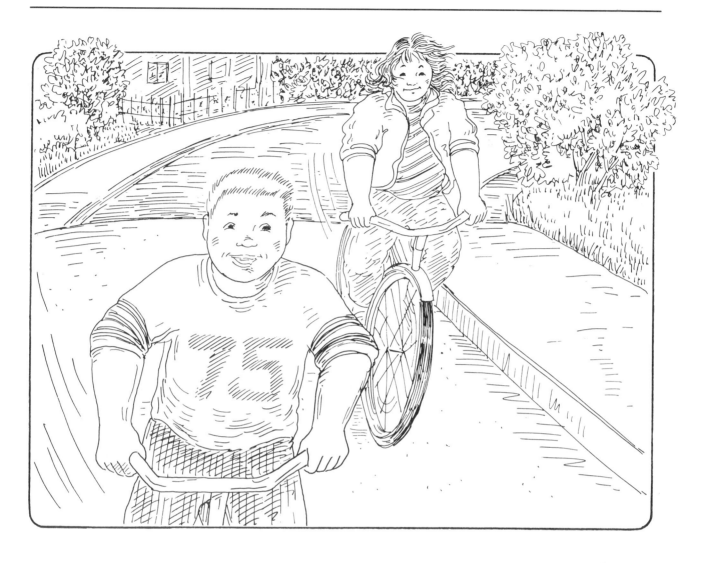

Next to the note was a crisp ten dollar bill.

Just as Cindy peeked over Matt's shoulder to read the note, he tore out of the house and hopped on his bike. Cindy picked up the ten dollar bill, climbed onto her bike and raced after Matt down the curvy street to the karate school with all the mirrors on the walls.

For the next hour she watched the karate master moan, yell and strike. Matt moved smoothly and swiftly. She loved it. Cindy wanted to try. The karate master brought her to the middle of the mat and showed her one move. She tried it and felt silly. She tried it again and still felt silly. By the tenth time Cindy got it right! Matt smiled. The karate master smiled. Finally, Cindy smiled.

Back on their bikes, they felt the cooling afternoon air whirr past their ears. They darted down the street then stopped abruptly at the corner grocery store.

They picked out fruit, checking each apple, orange and banana for bad spots and ripeness. Cindy picked out two firm peaches and three tangerines. They looked for non-fat yogurt and couldn't see any.

Cindy walked up to the lady behind the counter with thick brown glasses covered with dirt from the day's work, "Do you have any non-fat yogurt?"

The woman raised her left eyebrow almost to the top of her forehead. "Little girl, it's all non-fat yogurt. Can't you read?"

Cindy hung her head, slowly turned and walked to the back of the store. Now that she didn't get teased for being fat as much, she was being ridiculed for not reading. What luck!

Cindy said to Matt, who was reading the yogurt labels, "The checker lady with the brown glasses with two days worth of dirt on them says that they're all non-fat."

"Well," said Matt smugly, "some people don't know the difference between low-fat yogurt and non-fat yogurt."

Cindy smiled. She wasn't wrong after all. "Here's the non-fat yogurt, Matt, right on the bottom shelf! What do you want vanilla, peach or raspberry?"

"My Mom said vanilla, and she's the boss of the food we get, so let's get vanilla. I do like raspberry, so I'll ask her tonight during SHAPE-DOWN TIME if we could get raspberry next time."

Together Matt and Cindy marched up the aisle of the store with bags of fruit and cartons of vanilla non-fat yogurt, placed them on the counter and looked up at the checker lady. She quietly rang up their food — $6.15. Matt handed over the crisp ten dollar bill and she gave him back three quarters and three one dollar bills. He pocketed the change and picked up the brown paper bag brimming with fruit and yogurt.

"Wait!" said Cindy. The woman looked up sternly. "I mean, you owe us ten cents more, I think."

The woman's face softened. She took off her spotted, dusty glasses and said, "Pretty sharp, young lady. Here's your ten cents and an extra ten cents for being so alert."

Cindy blushed, clutched her two dimes and raced back to the bikes, not even noticing the racks of cookies and chips.

As Cindy and Matt slowly rode home, Cindy asked, "How'd I do, Matt?"

"You're a real champ, Cindy." he replied looking across his handlebars at her.

"I just wish my life was as exciting as yours. Can we trade lives, Matt, please?"

"Stick with your own life, Cindy. All we did was chores, exercise and interests. You can do that. You can start tomorrow. Just turn off the television. Pick out some things to do and do them!"

Cindy began to hum a sweet melody. Maybe she'd learn to play her grandpa's trumpet. Perhaps she'd ask her mom to sign her up for ballet lessons. Wouldn't it be fun to paint the fence in her front yard bright white? To race the vacuum around the downstairs rug? Her mind soared. Life was getting very, very exciting.

SMART TALK

Becoming active — Notice how your appetite changes? When you're doing something that's interesting and exciting, who cares about food? The hunger monster never knocks. Now, think again. What about when you come home from school to an empty house with nothing to do but homework? Microwaved pizza, chocolate chip cookies, even breakfast cereal and crackers beckon to you. Food surrounds you and convinces you that it's the only fun there is.

Food only helps hunger. It doesn't help you become stronger, smarter, more talented or better liked. Too much of it just makes you fatter. Television and food have one thing in common. They are both pacifiers. Imagine yourself with an oversized pacifier in your mouth every time you get hooked on television or food. Both television and food are good in small doses, but if they take up much time or attention they make a baby out of you.

So throw off those handcuffs of television and food and step into the world of activity. With activities you have to give a little more but you get a lot more back.

Think of a person stuck on television, food and school. That person grows up to be an adult who is stuck on television, food and work. Some life, huh? Now compare that to the

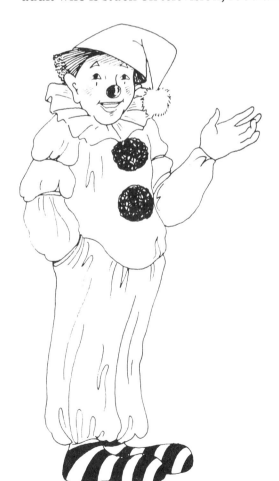

life you can build if you start doing things, begin learning how to keep up a home by doing chores, develop talents and interests with classes and activities, and train your body by learning sports or dance. Bingo! You're an adult. Look at your life! It's as varied as a rainbow. Food and television are only a small part of the pleasure you get from your exciting and fun life.

What is an active lifestyle? That's simple. For most children it's doing at least an hour of exercise, half an hour of chores and half an hour of enriching activities every day.

With your new active lifestyle you'll be doing exercise, chores and other activities every day. You'll be more independent, walking and biking more and taking care of the house. Instead of being the child who can't do anything, you'll be a member of the family who really helps out. And the bonus for you is that you don't have time for that bowl of chips and that stack of cookies. Food is not on your mind! And you feel so proud of yourself. Your parents feel so proud of you, too. You're their active, healthy kid!

YOUR TURN!

Cindy and Matt have started getting active! Pick out some of the things you'd like to do for chores and interests that scare away the boredom monster!

1. Check all of the things you could do at home:

_____ make your own bed

_____ clean up your own room

_____ fold your own laundry and put it away

_____ set the table

_____ clear the table

_____ wash/rinse dishes

_____ clean out dishwasher or dry/put away dishes

_____ wipe off counters

_____ dust tabletops

_____ help make fruit or veggie salads for dinner

_____ cook simple dinners

_____ take out the trash

_____ get the mail

_____ feed the dog/cat

_____ groom the dog/cat

_____ sweep the garage

_____ pull weeds

_____ water plants

_____ sort laundry and put it in the washer and dryer

_____ clean bathroom sink and bathtub

_____ buy a few things at the convenience store

_____ sweep and mop the floors

_____ vacuum

_____ bathe the dog

_____ walk the dog

_____ other:_____

2. Check all of the activities that interest you:

____ joining a sports team — like soccer	____ playing a musical instrument
____ taking a dance class — like ballet	____ joining a choir
____ taking gymnastics classes	____ going to the library
____ learning to play tennis	____ taking drama lessons
____ taking karate lessons	____ trying out for a play
____ learning to ski	____ building things from wood
____ learning to skate	____ sewing and needlework
____ arts and crafts	____ growing plants
____ collecting stamps	____ learning about animals
____ looking at stars	____ other_____
____ learning about space	

3. What do you think will happen to you if you become more active?

____ I won't feel bored as often.

____ I will have more fun.

____ I will learn how to do things.

____ I will be more independent.

____ I will eat less.

____ I will not watch as much television.

____ I will be happier.

____ other_____

STICKER STROKES

Check if I did it!

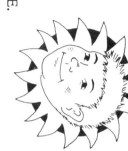

Each day I will:

	MON.	TUES.	WED.	THURS.	FRI.	SAT.	SUN.
Take SHAPEDOWN TIME.							
Write down my exercise.							
Eat at least one serving from each of the Four Food Groups for both lunch and dinner.							
Open up and tell someone how I feel.							
Exercise for 60 minutes or more.							
Watch no TV after I exercise, and limit TV to one hour.							
My choice: _____							

Number of goals I met:

My reward or privilege for making at least five goals every day this week is: _____ .

My weight: Start of the week _____   Goal _____   End of the week _____

98

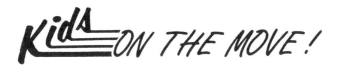

KidsON THE MOVE!

	MINUTES	ACTIVITY
MONDAY		
TUESDAY		
WEDNESDAY		
THURSDAY		
FRIDAY		
SATURDAY		
SUNDAY		

———JUST FOR FUN!———

WATCH TELEVISION!

Yes, watch television. For how long? A half hour per day. Watch your favorite kid's show and on Saturday and Sunday morning tune into cartoons.

Why watch television?

To analyze the food commercials. In one year the average kid watches between 8,500 and 13,000 food and beverage commercials. The people who make the commercials are paid 400 to 600 million dollars a year just to bring food and drink messages to kids like you. They want you to buy their product. They're not concerned with how their food or beverage affects your health, your teeth or your weight. Their job is to trick, sweet-talk and excite you into wanting their product.

They do convince some kids to want JUNK FOOD, to ask their parents for JUNK FOOD and to eat JUNK FOOD. Do you want to do what the advertisers say to do? Do you want advertising messages to seep into your brain and coax you to eat foods that do your body no good?

Check commercials

Name the food or drink you saw advertised in each of the ways listed below. Which of these ways did they use to try to make you want their food or drink? When you look at commercials, watch the people. Listen to the music. See what people are doing. Pay attention to the words they use. Write in the name of the food or drink that used these techniques.

1. The same characters that are on the show are on the commercial. (The message: The characters you like recommend our product.)

    Food or drink_____

2. The people look normal weight and healthy even though they are eating sugary, fatty foods. (The message: You can eat lots of sugary, fatty foods and still be healthy and look great.)

    Food or drink_____

3. They say it's super nutritious even though it contains lots of salt (like soup), fat (like cheese) or sugar (like granola bars).

    Food or drink_____

JUST FOR FUN!

4. They use a famous person or cartoon character in the commercial. (The message: "If you like this person, you'll like this food or drink.)

   Food or drink_____

5. They do exciting things in the commercial like downhill skiing, windsurfing or swimming. (The message: "If you buy this food or drink you're life will be fun and exciting.")

   Food or drink_____

6. They surround the person with people who love or admire him or her. (The message is "You'll be popular and loved if you buy this product!")

   Food or drink_____

Do these ways of tricking, sweet-talking and exciting you work? Will you buy these six products?

      yes   sometimes   no

9. AMY LEARNS A LESSON

Tomorrow would be Jesse's birthday. The other three kids in the cozy corner of Ms. Bacon's class were planning a party for him. Everybody knew about it, that is, except Jesse. Amy, Cindy and Matt had invited the whole class to meet right after school near the tall trees next to the library for the party.

Ms. Baker knew about it and said that she would bring the plates, cups, table cloths and napkins. She even said that she would bring her baby birds to class that day to add to the festivities! Sophia at the office knew, too. She said she'd hope for clear skies and bright sunshine for that afternoon.

With only one day to go Amy, Cindy and Matt gathered together at the corner table in the lunch area to plan the party.

"Let's play soccer," suggested Cindy.

"Good idea! That's Jesse's favorite sport!" responded Matt.

"What about music?" asked Cindy.

"I know. I'll bring my tape player," volunteered Amy.

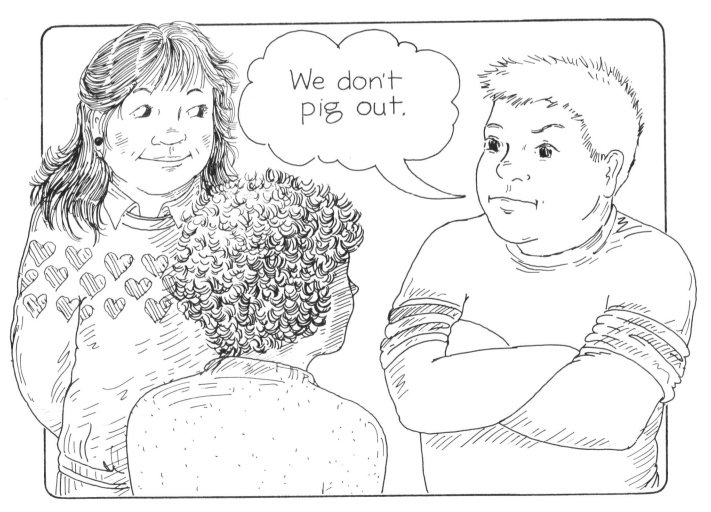

"And I'll bring my tapes," said both Matt and Cindy in unison.

"Great!" replied Amy.

There was silence.

"Ummm. What about food, Matt?" asked Cindy.

"Why, of course, we'll have chocolate fudge cake topped with miniature marshmallows. It's my favorite," interrupted Amy.

Matt looked at Cindy. Cindy looked at Matt.

Slowly Matt said, "Good idea, Amy. Why don't you bring that since it's your favorite?"

Cindy continued, "But not everybody wants to eat greasy, gooey cake so I'll bring a fruit salad."

"And I'll bring a plate of veggies with my favorite dip," said Matt.

"Veggies? Who wants to eat veggies at a party? This is supposed to be fun, you know," snarled Amy.

Matt snickered softly and turned to Amy, "I'm sure, Amy, that we can all have fun whether we're stuffing our faces with gooey chocolate marshmallow cake, crunching on crisp veggies or slurping up mounds of cut-up fruit. The party and the people are the fun, not the goop!"

Cindy winked at Matt. If only Clown could see Matt now!

"Remember Valentine's Day, Amy?" said Cindy.

"Sure I do. I had the flu and my dad brought me a huge red heart with chocolate and marsh-mallow creams in it."

"Did the creams make your Valentine's Day happy?" probed Matt.

"My Valentine's Day wasn't very happy anyway. My nose was drippy and my head ached. I almost had to go to the doctor's."

"What about the creams?" asked Cindy.

"They were pretty, but they didn't taste very good. They were under my bed until last week when an army of ants got them." Amy explained.

"For Valentine's Day my mom gave me a mystery book for my collection and my grandpa gave me a red rose. We all went to a movie together," said Cindy.

"We had fun, too. My mom and dad gave me a new professional football and we went to the school field and played touch football with our neighbor. It was crisp and cold but we ran so much that we were sweating! It was a great day!"

"You guys are making me feel dumb," said Amy, pouting.

"We're not making you feel any way. Besides, how can you feel dumb when you have the best math grades in the whole class? We're just telling you how we celebrate holidays and parties. We don't pig out," said Matt.

"Okay," challenged Amy, "you don't pig out at birthday parties or Valentine's Day, but what about Halloween and Christmas? I bet you crawl on your knees to get candy and cookies then!"

Cindy smiled at her friend and gently put her arm around her, "No, Amy, the fun of Halloween is the costumes and the parties. I'll still get

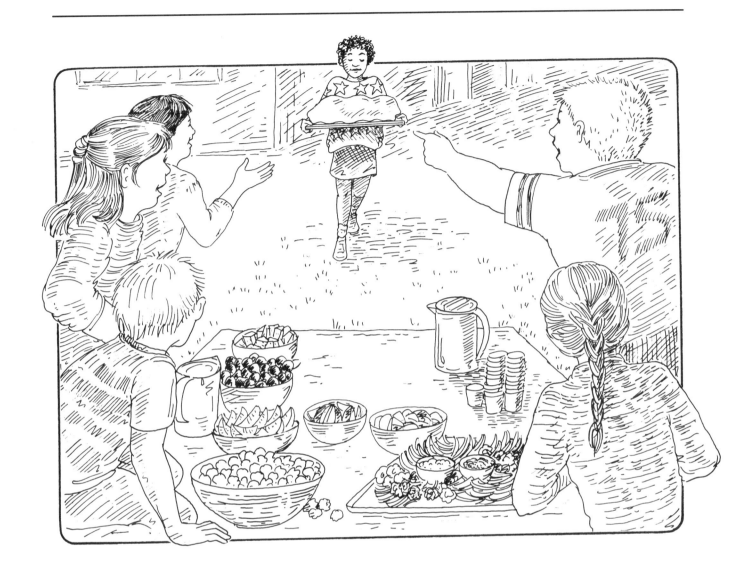

some candy this year, but I probably won't eat much of it."

Matt added, "The holidays may be a little harder, but even if I'm surrounded by cookies, I eat some of them but I won't stuff them in."

Amy raised her eyebrow, "You won't? How come? Is it because you can't because you're still a little chunky?"

"That's not it. Some of that stuff is okay even when I'm losing weight. It's just that I don't crave it any more. I can get it when I want it and that's enough. I don't eat a lot of candy and cookies because I've stopped wanting them. I'm more interested in things other than eating."

"I bet you don't have six cavities every year when you go to the dentist like I do," sighed Amy.

Matt and Cindy smiled and Cindy turned to Amy, "One year I had 10 cavities. This year I'm shooting for none!"

The next day was Jesse's party. Sophia's wishes paid off. The day was bright and sunny with a light breeze that lifted the spirits. Ms. Bacon brought her birds and the kids peeked at them one at a time. Ms. Bacon said that the birds were very sensitive and couldn't tolerate too much noise and stimulation. She gave the biggest baby bird to Jesse for his birthday. He could pick it up as soon as the baby bird was ready to leave his mother.

When the last bell rang at school, all the kids in Ms. Bacon's class, including all four children in the cozy corner, sprang for the door and raced to the grove of trees next to the library. Out of the backpacks sprang party food. Cindy brought cut up pears, peaches, apples, oranges and pineapple. Matt uncovered a huge tray of carrots, celery, cucumbers, broccoli and radishes all cut up, and two bowls of dip. They laid them all out on the tablecloth that Ms. Bacon had brought.

Where was Amy's chocolate fudge cake with miniature marshmallows on top? In fact, where was Amy? Cindy and Matt looked all around.

"There she is!" shouted Matt, "over there, coming from the office." Amy walked toward them carrying a large platter covered with a cloth. She took each step carefully. All the kids began to gather around the tablecloth, helping themselves to veggies and fruit and waiting for Amy to unveil her cake.

Amy walked up to the group and gently placed the platter in the middle of the tablecloth. It was warm. It smelled wonderful and fresh.

"Jesse," called Cindy, "come quickly!"

Jesse raced to the tablecloth and fell to his knees. Amy smiled at him and lifted the cloth.

Fresh bread! Fragrant, soft whole wheat bread! Five loaves of it with candles stuck in each—11 candles altogether.

"Bread?" said David.

"Bread?" said Jesse.

"That's right, it's bread!" said Amy.

Just then the aroma of the fresh bread swirled around them and Cindy threw her head back,

breathed in and said, "Ohhhhhh! It smells so wonderful!"

"Mmmmm," said David, "It smells almost as good as cake."

Amy gloated and turned as Sophia began cutting the fresh bread, "I brought the dough to school and Sophia helped me bake it in the school oven."

Jesse reached for a piece of bread and bit into a soft fragrant slice still warm from the oven. "It's not cake, but it's delicious!"

The rest of the kids from Ms. Bacon's room 6 each grabbed a piece of bread and took off for the soccer field. Later, after the birthday songs had been sung, the veggies crunched, the fruit salad slurped, the bread munched, and the tablecloths, plates and napkins cleaned up, Cindy and Matt talked as they slowly walked home. They had joined their SHAPEDOWN CLUB 10 weeks ago. The group was winding down, even though they would go see the group leader every so often.

Cindy felt sad. "I'm going to miss the kids in the group, Matt, especially Kristin and Michael."

"And I'm going to miss Jason and Ben. I wish they went to our school," said Matt.

"Yes, but we can still be SHAPEDOWN buddies, can't we?" asked Cindy.

"Of course we can, Cindy," replied Matt. "Plus we have another special friend to count on."

"Me?" questioned Clown appearing on the stone wall next to the sidewalk.

Cindy laughed, "Clown, I've been meaning to give you a hug!" and she reached over to give him a very warm hug with her not so round, not so soft and not so fluffy body.

Matt stayed back. "Clown," he said seriously, "You've helped me a lot, too. See my body? It's a little leaner. And I've stopped stuffing and starving. I have a ways to go until I need smaller pants, but I'm getting there!"

Cindy let Clown out of her warm embrace, "And you've helped me talk about my feelings and stand up for myself. Sure I'm getting leaner, but I'm also happier and busier. I don't even have much time for television anymore." Cindy turned to Matt, "And you, too, my buddy. You've helped me every step of the way."

Matt smiled, "We've been good buddies for each other, alright, but I'm worried I won't keep it up!"

Clown stepped forward, his suit filled out with muscles and vitality, "I'm not worried much. Ups and downs are normal. When my eating and exercise aren't healthy, it's no big deal. I haven't blown it. I've just taken a little vacation from healthy habits. I'm just going to get right back on track."

"That's right, Matt," interjected Cindy. "Plus we can still visit our group leader whenever we want. That will help us get back on track. And we can talk with our families. They'll help, too."

Cindy turned on her heels and with a wink and a smile shouted, "Hey, you two, race you to my house!"

Matt and Cindy raced down the street and streaked around the corner. Clown disappeared from the rock wall and reappeared on the counter in Cindy's kitchen. Like magic he folded up his legs, making himself into a cookie jar once again. He heard the door bang as Cindy and Matt came running in, still laughing. There was a little bit of magic in the air that didn't come from Clown. It came from two other smart people, Matt and Cindy.

SMART TALK

Special occasions—Birthdays, Valentine's Day, Halloween, Christmas or Hanukkah, Easter, and Thanksgiving are festive times. They usually mean JUNK FOOD. But eating is only part of the fun. You can have a great time without overeating. What can you do to make special occasions fun yet healthy?

Ask your mom and dad to stop giving you food gifts. Tell them you want flowers, money, books, toys or anything else that isn't food.

If you get food gifts, give them away. Food gifts are fun to look at and play with, but they won't help you become leaner and fitter. If you like, have a taste or two, then give it away.

Ask your mom and dad to serve more veggies, fruits and other lighter foods for holidays and parties.

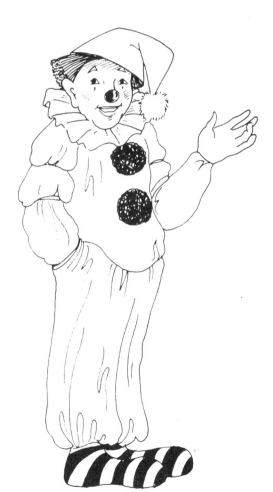

Praise your mom and dad when they serve lighter foods or give you things other than food. Moms and dads like praise, too.

Before a party, during SHAPEDOWN TIME, plan what you will eat at the party. If you want to eat sweet or fatty foods, plan trade-offs so that parties don't stop you from losing weight.

Speak up and say "no thanks" when food you didn't plan to eat is offered to you.

Keep in mind that the fun of parties is mainly the people and activities—not the food. Halloween is fun because you have costumes, parties and trick or treating. You also get to sort and play with the candy. Is eating the candy really the best part of the holiday? Most kids say "NO!"

You have done well! In the last few weeks you have made some changes in your food and exercise. You have probably made some changes in your fitness and weight, too. You know more about nutrition, exercise and communication. Chances are your family has made some healthy changes, too.

SMART TALK continued

This part of SHAPEDOWN is coming to an end. You can plan what kind of help you want during the coming weeks to keep up the healthy habits you have started in SHAPEDOWN.

Most families continue to get help from their SHAPEDOWN group leader. You may want to see him or her weekly or monthly for the next year as you go through ups and downs of making your food and exercise habits stick. Keep track of your weight by weighing once a week. You and your family will plan to take SHAPEDOWN TIME either every night or just once a week.

The changes you have started in SHAPEDOWN will not disappear. They are not magic. They are better than magic. They are real. You have learned to talk about your feelings and needs, to eat in a healthy way, and to enjoy exercise more. You have made these changes. Nobody made them for you. Now it's your job to continue them. When the going gets tough, it's your job to ask for some help from your parent or group leader.

When you get off track and stop exercising and eating well, it's not the end of the world. You're just taking a little vacation from healthy habits. The trick is to get back to exercising and eating well right away.

Thanks for being part of SHAPEDOWN. It's not easy to have a weight problem as a kid. But there are some good things about it. You can use the ideas you learned in SHAPEDOWN with lots of problems — not just weight. So you have a head start on other kids in knowing how to handle difficulties like a pro.

You've also helped your family shape up their food and exercise. We hope SHAPEDOWN has helped them feel healthier and closer and that it has given you the boost you needed to put weight problems behind you and get on with a more fun and active life.

YOUR TURN!

1. Cindy has started getting her party fun from people, not food. Matt has asked his mom to stop giving him candy gifts. Name one fun thing that doesn't involve food about each of these special occasions.

Valentine's Day _____

Halloween _____

Thanksgiving _____

Christmas/Hanukkah _____

Birthday parties _____

2. List the special occasions or holidays for which your parents or other people give you food gifts (candy and other sweets).

the occasion   the food they give me

_____   _____

_____   _____

_____   _____

3. Ask your parents or these other people to stop giving you food gifts. Tell them what gifts you would like instead of food. Check the gifts you would like:

____ flowers   ____ movie tickets

____ books   ____ a friend overnight

____ games   ____ a new toy

____ balls   ____ clothes

____ money   ____ jewelry

____ family outing   ____ other things_____

____ an outing with a friend

4. Ask you Mom and Dad to serve lighter foods for special occasions and holidays. Check the foods you'd like them to serve as part of special occasion meals:

____ veggies and dip	____ light ice cream
____ bread sticks	____ sugar-free sodas
____ fresh fruit salad	____ mineral water and fruit juice
____ crisp salads	____ veggies without fat
____ bread without butter	____ rice or potatoes without fat
____ fruit desserts	

5. Which of these changes did you make in SHAPEDOWN?

____ know more about food and exercise	____ do more chores
____ talk about my feelings more	____ communicate better with my parents
____ speak up about my needs and problems more	____ family feels closer
____ exercise more	____ feel better about my body
____ eat more regular meals	____ feel better about me
____ eat more LIGHT FOODS and FREE FOODS	____ am stronger
____ eat less	____ am more flexible
____ any more active after school	____ can run farther before I get tired
____ have more interests and activities	____ lost weight
	____ other_____

6. Look at your FOOD SUMMARY at the end of this book. Pick three FREE FOODS that you don't usually eat to eat this week. They are your TARGET FREE FOODS.

1._____

2._____

3._____

7. Pick three JUNK FOODS that you still eat. They are your TARGET JUNK FOODS. Do not eat them this week.

1._____

2._____

3._____

8. What are your goals for the next three months?

I will lose weight: _____ pounds

I will exercise more: _____ minutes

          _____ days per week

Kinds of exercise:_____

_____

_____

I will eat better: _____ eat more FREE FOODS and LIGHT FOODS

      _____ at breakfast

      _____ at lunch

      _____ at dinner

      _____ at snack

      _____ I will eat less

I will speak up more: _____ about my feelings

      _____ about my needs

      _____ about my thoughts

      _____ about my problems

I will feel better: _____ about myself

      _____ about my body

Other goals: _____

_____

_____

9. What kinds of help do you want in the next three months?

____ SHAPEDOWN TIME:

every night   once a week   when we need it   other_____

____ Family weigh-in:

once a week   other_____

____ Visits to my SHAPEDOWN group leader:

weekly   every other week   once a month   other_____

____ Other kinds of help_____

Thank you!

STICKER STROKES   Check if I did it!

	MON.	TUES.	WED.	THURS.	FRI.	SAT.	SUN.

Each day I will:

Take SHAPEDOWN TIME.

Write down what I eat for dinner through bed time.

Eat at least one of my **TARGET FREE FOODS.**

Not eat my **TARGET JUNK FOODS.**

Exercise for 60 minutes or more.

Watch no TV until after I exercise, and limit TV to one hour.

My choice: _____

Number of goals I met: — — — — — — —

My reward or privilege for making at least five goals every day this week is: _____

My weight:

Start of the week _____   End of the week _____

Goal _____

114

MY DINNER

MONDAY	
TUESDAY	
WEDNESDAY	
THURSDAY	
FRIDAY	
SATURDAY	
SUNDAY	

Number of days I had mainly FREE FOODS and LIGHT FOODS_____

Number of days I ate foods from all of the Four Food Groups_____

JUST FOR FUN!

MAKE PIZZA!

You love pizza, right? Right. Then make it. Pizza is fun to make and eat! Your tummy stands up and applauds and your tongue dances the jig when pizza is in town.

But isn't pizza a heavy food? That depends. Ever had a greasy pizza with pounds of cheese and bubbles of fat on top from the salami, pepperoni and sausage? That's definitely heavy. You know it's heavy from tasting the grease and from feeling the lead in your stomach afterwards.

But pizza can be light, too. Take the pizza you'll make this week—lots of whole wheat bread for the crust, some spicy tomato sauce, a sprinkling of cheese and the crunch of vegetables.

Gather these things:

frozen wheat bread dough

a jar of pizza sauce

mozarella cheese—reduced fat

two or more veggies: mushrooms, green peppers, onions, green onions, zucchini, garlic, tomatoes

Create your own pizza:

5 to 7 hours before serving:

1. Take one loaf of bread dough out of the freezer.
2. Put it into a bowl and cover it with a towel.
3. Put the bowl in a warm (not hot!) place for 4 to 6 hours until it has thawed and has doubled in size.
4. Grate mozzarella cheese until you have one cup of it.
5. Chop and slice 2 cups of vegetables

JUST FOR FUN!

1 hour before serving:

1. Preheat oven 350 degrees
2. Punch down the dough with your fist (punch, punch, punch).
3. Roll the dough out on a floured board to form a 12-inch circle.
4. Place the dough on a non-stick pan.
5. Top the dough with a cup of pizza sauce, cheese and veggies.
6. Bake for 20 to 30 minutes until bubbling and browned.

Enjoy your pizza!

Set the table for a prince or princess. Someone important will eat the pizza—you! Put out placemats and napkins and turn off the television. Serve up the pizza and slowly enjoy each and every bite.

Which vegetables did you put on top of your pizza?

_____

Rate your own cooking. How did your pizza taste?

     bad   okay   good

     1   2   3   4   5

MY BODY

	Date ___/___/___	Date ___/___/___	Date ___/___/___
Weight (pounds)			
Height (inches)			
Triceps skinfold (mm)			
Waist circumference (inches)			
Hip circumference (inches)			
Waist:hip ratio			
Blood Pressure	___/___	___/___	___/___
Strength: curl-ups (# in 1 min.)			
Flexibility: sit and reach (inches)			
Endurance: step test (min./sec. up to 3/0)	___/___	___/___	___/___
step test (1 min. heart rate)			

MY WEIGHT RECORD

Write down your weight. This weight corresponds to the "0" at the far left under week 1. See the black dot at that point. Compare your weight each week with your starting weight. Plot it accordingly. For example, if your starting weight was 162 pounds and your weight at week 2 was 161 pounds, you should put a dot a −1 under week 2. Then connect the two dots. Continue plotting your weight like this each week.

MY STARTING WEIGHT:_____   MY ENDING WEIGHT:_____

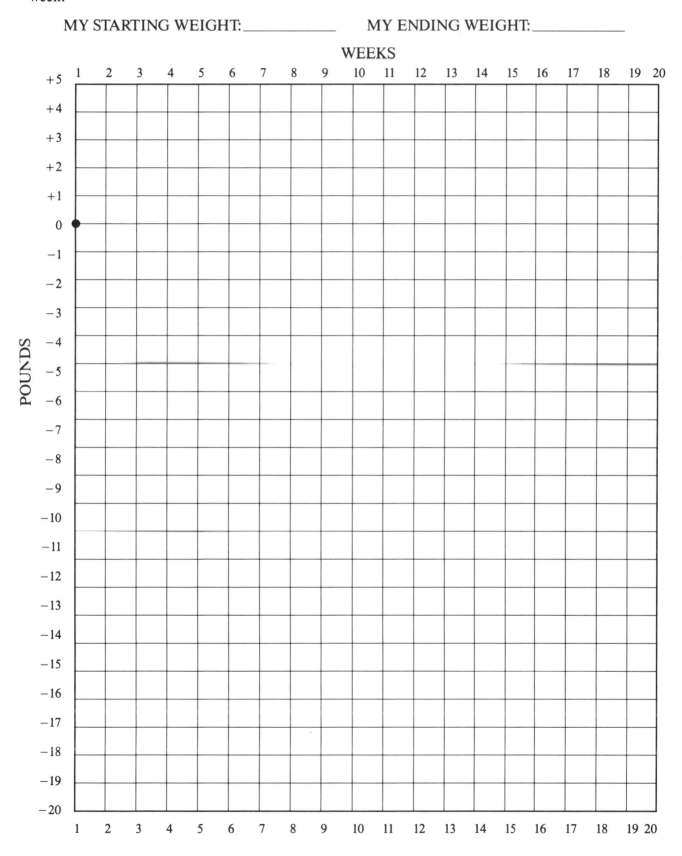

FOOD SUMMARY

FREE FOODS

artichokes	greens	water chestnuts	plain popcorn
asparagus	jicama	zucchini	tabasco sauce
bamboo shoots	lettuce	water	soy sauce
broccoli	mushrooms	mineral water	horseradish
brussels sprouts	onions	diet soda	garlic
cabbage	peppers	soda water	onion powder
carrots	radishes	tea	cinnamon
cauliflower	sauerkraut	coffee	herbs
celery	sour pickles	broth	spices
cucumbers	dill pickles	tomato juice	flavorings
eggplant	sprouts	vegetable juice	mustard
green beans	summer squash	limes	vinegar
green onions	tomatoes	lemons	no-oil salad dressing

LIGHT FOODS

non-fat milk	fish	papaya	clear soups
low-fat milk (1%)	tuna, canned	pineapple	vegetable soups
non-fat buttermilk	in water	peaches	bread
reduced fat cheese	lean red meat,	plums	bread sticks
low-fat cottage	all fat removed	raisins	biscuits
cheese	apples	prunes	english muffins
plain low-fat	applesauce, canned	strawberries	hamburger buns
yogurt	without sugar	tangerines	low-fat crackers
dried beans	apricots	watermelons	unsweetened cereal
split peas	bananas	fruit, canned	hominy grits
black-eyed peas	blackberries	in water	tortillas
lentils	cantaloupe	fruit, canned	plain spaghetti
refried beans	cherries	in juice	rice cakes
turkey, light	grapefruit	potatoes	rice
meat, no skin	grapes	sweet potatoes	bran
chicken, light	nectarines	peas	barley
meat, no skin	oranges	winter squash	bulgar

HEAVY FOODS

low-fat milk (2%)	almonds	cream soups	coconut
whole milk	sunflower seeds	macaroni &	fries
chocolate milk	chicken or turkey	cheese	hash browns
cheese	with skin	macaroni salad	sweetened cereals
creamed cottage	chicken or turkey	potato salad	granola
cheese	dark meat	pizza	high-fat crackers
flavored yogurt	fried chicken	chili	taco shells
ice milk	turkey hot dogs	avocado	stuffing
low-fat frozen	fish sticks	sauced vegetables	corn bread
yogurt	fried fish	fruit rolls	muffins
pudding	tuna, packed in	sweetened	pancakes
tofu	oil	applesauce	waffles
peanuts	red meat	fruit, canned	french toast
peanut butter	eggs	in syrup	buttered popcorn

JUNK FOODS

ice cream	fruit drinks	candy	beer
sherbet	kool-aid	chocolate	wine
shakes	jello	chocolate topping	liquor
cream cheese	chips	syrup	butter
sour cream	pies	honey	margarine
half and half	cakes	jam	oil
whipped cream	cookies	jelly	lard
cream sauce	doughnuts	marmalade	gravy
bacon	pastries	sugar	mayonnaise
sausage	croissants	popsicles	tartar sauce
hot dogs	candy cereal	regular sodas	salad dressing
salami	granola candy	sweet pickles	olives
salt pork	bars	gum	salt